Weekly iron and folic acid supplementation programmes for women of reproductive age

An analysis of best programme practices

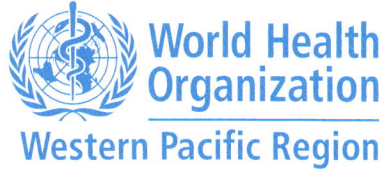

WHO Library Cataloguing in Publication Data

Weekly iron and folic acid supplementation programmes for women of reproductive age: An analysis of best programme practices

1. Anaemia, Iron-Deficiency–prevention and control. 2. Iron. 3. Folic acid. 4. Dietary supplements. 5. Women's health.

ISBN 978 92 9061 523 1   (NLM Classification: WA 309)

© World Health Organization 2011

All rights reserved. Publications of the World Health Organization can be obtained from WHO Press, World Health Organization, 20 Avenue Appia, 1211 Geneva 27, Switzerland (tel.: +41 22 791 3264; fax: +41 22 791 4857; e-mail: bookorders@who.int). Requests for permission to reproduce or translate WHO publications – whether for sale or for noncommercial distribution – should be addressed to WHO Press, at the above address (fax: +41 22 791 4806; e-mail: permissions@who.int). For WHO Western Pacific Regional Publications, request for permission to reproduce should be addressed to the Publications Office, World Health Organization, Regional Office for the Western Pacific, P.O. Box 2932, 1000, Manila, Philippines, (fax: +632 521 1036, e-mail: publications@wpro.who.int).

The designations employed and the presentation of the material in this publication do not imply the expression of any opinion whatsoever on the part of the World Health Organization concerning the legal status of any country, territory, city or area or of its authorities, or concerning the delimitation of its frontiers or boundaries. Dotted lines on maps represent approximate border lines for which there may not yet be full agreement.

The mention of specific companies or of certain manufacturers' products does not imply that they are endorsed or recommended by the World Health Organization in preference to others of a similar nature that are not mentioned. Errors and omissions excepted, the names of proprietary products are distinguished by initial capital letters.

All reasonable precautions have been taken by the World Health Organization to verify the information contained in this publication. However, the published material is being distributed without warranty of any kind, either expressed or implied. The responsibility for the interpretation and use of the material lies with the reader. In no event shall the World Health Organization be liable for damages arising from its use.

Table of Contents

Acknowledgements	iv
Executive Summary	1

Section I : Background, objectives and methodology — 5

Section II : Global WIFS programmes for WRA — an analysis — 9

    Section II A: Key findings and observations — 10

    Section II B: Best programme practices — 17

Section III : WIFS programmes — Country case studies — 35

    1. India (Bihar) — 36

    2. India (Gujarat) — 45

    3. India (Madhya Pradesh) — 56

    4. India (Uttar Pradesh) — 64

    5. Egypt — 76

    6. The Lao People's Democratic Republic — 87

    7. Viet Nam (Yen Bai Province) — 98

    8. Viet Nam (Hai Duong Province) — 108

    9. Cambodia — 119

    10. The Philippines — 131

Annexes — 143

    Annex 1 : Documentation of process and impact of selected case studies on preventive weekly IFA supplementation (WIFS) for women of reproductive age (WRA) — 144

    Annex 2 : The Recommendations of the WHO Global Expert Consultation on Weekly Iron and Folic Acid Supplementation for Preventing Anaemia in Women of Reproductive Age — 148

    Annex 3 : Criteria for ensuring the quality of iron and folic acid supplement tablets — 154

    Annex 4 : Indicators for establishing, monitoring and evaluating programmes — 155

Acknowledgements

This study was undertaken and documented for the WHO Regional Office for the Western Pacific by Dr Sheila C. Vir (WHO Consultant) and Dr L.T. Cavalli-Sforza (Regional Adviser in Nutrition, WHO Regional Office for the Western Pacific). Expert comments were provided by Dr Suttalik Smitasiri and Dr Usha Ramakrishnan. Sincere thanks are due to Dr Fernando E. Viteri for his interest, encouragement and support.

The authors are grateful to the following, who completed the template and responded to innumerable queries: Dr Bounthom Phengdy (Lao People's Democratic Republic), Dr Gerard J. Casey (Melbourne, Australia), Dr Beverly Ann Biggs (Melbourne, Australia), Ms La-Ong Tokmoh, (Cambodia), Dr Nagwa El Ashry (Egypt) , Dr Ayoub Eid Aljawaldeh (WHO Egypt), Dr Mohamed Ayoya (India), DrNeelam Singh (Uttar Pradesh, India), Dr Farhat Saiyed (Bihar, India), Dr Vandana Aggarwal (Madhya Pradesh, India), Dr Narayan Gaonkar and Ms Purvi D. Karkar (Gujarat, India). The authors also greatly appreciate the support of Ms Ritu Jain (Research Nutritionist, Public Health Nutrition and Development Centre, New Delhi, India) for her statistical support.

The comments on the final draft received from the following experts were extremely useful and their contributions are appreciated: Dr Barbara Underwood, Dr Fernando Viteri, Dr Ian Darnton Hill, Dr Lynnette M. Nuefeld, Dr Deepika Chaudhery, Dr Anand Lakshman, Dr Viviana Mangiaterra, Dr Nancy Haselow, Dr Akoto Osei, Dr Mary Dunbar, Dr Narimah Awin, Dr Judy Mclean, Dr Gerard John Casey, Dr Ornello Lincetto and Dr Suttliak Smitasiri.

We would like to thank Danxi Cheng for her careful final editing of the document.

The World Health Organization gratefully acknowledges the financial contribution of the Ministry of Health, Labour and Welfare, Japan towards the completion of this publication.

Executive Summary

What is the issue?

In a developing country, the provision of weekly iron and folic acid supplements (WIFS) to women of reproductive age (WRA) should be viewed as a key intervention to prevent anaemia and improve folate status.

Globally, 1.62 billion people are anaemic, many due to iron deficiency[1]. One out of three WRA is estimated to be anaemic[2]. Non-pregnant women are the population group with the greatest number of individuals affected by anaemia (468.4 million)[1]. The consequences of iron deficiency, particularly for WRA, are far-reaching. Iron deficiency contributes to maternal mortality, foetal growth retardation and perinatal mortality. Research has shown that improving iron and folate nutrition, not only influences safe motherhood and birth outcomes, but also enhances the health and well-being of WRA by optimizing educational performance and increasing overall productivity.

Unfortunately, past approaches have not been effective in preventing and controlling iron deficiency and anaemia. The WHO Global Consultation on Weekly Iron and Folic Acid Supplementation for Preventing Anaemia in Women of Reproductive Age (April 2007) therefore reached the consensus that critical elements of WIFS programmes must be identified to ensure the successful implementation of such programmes worldwide and, ultimately, to improve the iron status of WRA and reduce the prevalence of anaemia. A study was therefore undertaken in 2008–2009 with the objective of identifying best programme practices for planning and implementation of WIFS programmes.

It is envisaged that the information on critical programme elements and practices drawn together in this document will serve to support advocacy, accelerate planning and strengthen implementation of WIFS programmes for WRA by programme planners and managers.

How was information gathered?

The first step of the study involved defining the criteria for selection of WIFS programmes for WRA. Based on the agreed criteria, 10 programmes were identified. A standard template was used to gather programme information and document case studies. These case studies were analysed in terms of:

- strategy;
- intervention package;
- critical programme components, including type of IFA supplements used; and
- innovative, effective actions for improving compliance.

---

1 *World prevalence of anaemia 1993-2005.*, World Health Organization, Geneva, 2008.

2 McLean E, *et al.* Worldwide prevalence of anaemia in preschool aged children, pregnant women and non-pregnant women of reproductive age In: Kraemer K, Zimmermann MB, eds. *Nutritional anemia.* Sight and Life Press, 2007.

Lessons learnt were summarized and best programme practices were extracted.

A major constraint in the study was the fact that the process documentation was often incomplete. This resulted in intensive follow-up with implementers to fill in the gaps, and made the documentation of case studies a complex exercise.

A total of 10 programmes across six countries were identified: two from Viet Nam, four from India and the remaining four from Cambodia, Egypt, the Lao People's Democratic Republic and the Philippines. In five of the programmes, the target group included WRA. In all the programmes, except one in Viet Nam, the target population also included adolescent girls, both in and out of school. The WIFS programme to include both adolescent boys and girls.

Two distinct programme processes were used:

1. free supply of WIFS to WRA, accompanied by nutrition education; and
2. selling of iron-folic acid (IFA) supplements to WRA using a social marketing approach.

Seven programmes utilized the first process, with Cambodia, the Philippines and Hai Duong Province in Viet Nam using the second strategy.

WIFS tablets used across the programmes varied in composition. Elemental iron content was either 60 mg or 100 mg, while folic acid content ranged from 0.3 to 3.5 mg. No rationale was presented regarding the selection of composition for the supplement; generally, however, the lower doses of folic acid corresponded to those found in daily iron/folic acid supplements, which were used in some projects as weekly supplements, while the higher dose (3.5 mg) was used in Cambodia, the Lao People's Democratic Republic, the Philippines and Viet Nam based on previous efficacy studies aimed at providing folic acid supplementation sufficient for one week. Cost varied from US$0.12 to $3.64 for an annual supply of 52 IFA supplements. The delivery channels for WIFS were not limited to the health sector but also included schools, institutions, factories and women's groups; in Cambodia, the Ministry of Women's Affairs and Ministry of Education, Youth and Sport were also involved. Biannual administration of deworming was undertaken in seven of the 10 programmes. Over a period of 6-16 months, there was wide variation in the reduction of anaemia prevalence, ranging from 8.9% to 56.8%. Compliance in taking the WIFS was about 70% or greater in all WIFS programmes except one.

What strategies were effective in supporting women to take WIFS?

The programme practice of fixing one day in the week as "WIFS Day" or "Iron Day" to promote consumption of WIFS was universal. That strategy addressed the problem of "forgetfulness", a primary factor adversely influencing compliance. Adverse side-effects of WIFS were low, between 5% to 20%, and therefore had little impact on compliance. Promoting consumption of IFA on a full stomach before retiring at night further contributed to addressing the issue of adverse side-effects. However, it should be noted that consumption of iron near a meal reduces iron absorption, and this may be partly responsible for a lower reduction in anaemia rates observed in some projects. Taking the supplements at least two hours after a meal, before retiring at night, is considered the best option.

A communication strategy emphasizing the benefits of WIFS experienced by WRA, rather than the side-effects, played a positive role in creating demand for WIFS and increasing compliance. Health and nutrition education, as well as social marketing strategies, often based on formative research, along with advocacy and social mobilization activities, improved acceptance of iron supplementation. Establishing a simple and user-friendly monitoring system played a critical role in modifying programme design and sustaining the improved compliance rate. Individual self-monitoring or institution-based monitoring was considered practical, feasible and effective. Investing in supervision during WIFS consumption was not feasible and provided no added value compared with monitoring.

What information does this study contain?

The WIFS programme practices emerging from the analysis of the programmes reviewed are presented in Section II of the document, while Section III presents the case studies of the 10 WIFS programmes. Section IIB highlights details of best programme practices with reference to target populations and strategies for accessing IFA supplements. It also provides information on delivery mechanisms for IFA supplements, critical elements of communication strategies, actions for improving compliance, user-friendly monitoring systems and the principles followed for capacity development.

What solutions does this study propose?

This study proposes the use of a two-pronged approach in developing countries for improvement of iron nutrition and prevention of iron deficiency anaemia:

- free WIFS supply accompanied by nutrition education for socioeconomically disadvantaged groups; and
- investment in social marketing of WIFS to WRA who have the resources to purchase low-cost IFA supplements.

For a brief synopsis of the 10 best practice interventions, please refer to *'Best practice top 10'*, which appears in *Weekly iron and folic acid supplementation programmes for women of reproductive age: an analysis of best programme practices (short version)*. Manila, World Health Organization Regional Office for the Western Pacific, 2011. See also the WHO WPRO website: http://www.wpro.who.int/health_topics/nutrition/publications.htm.

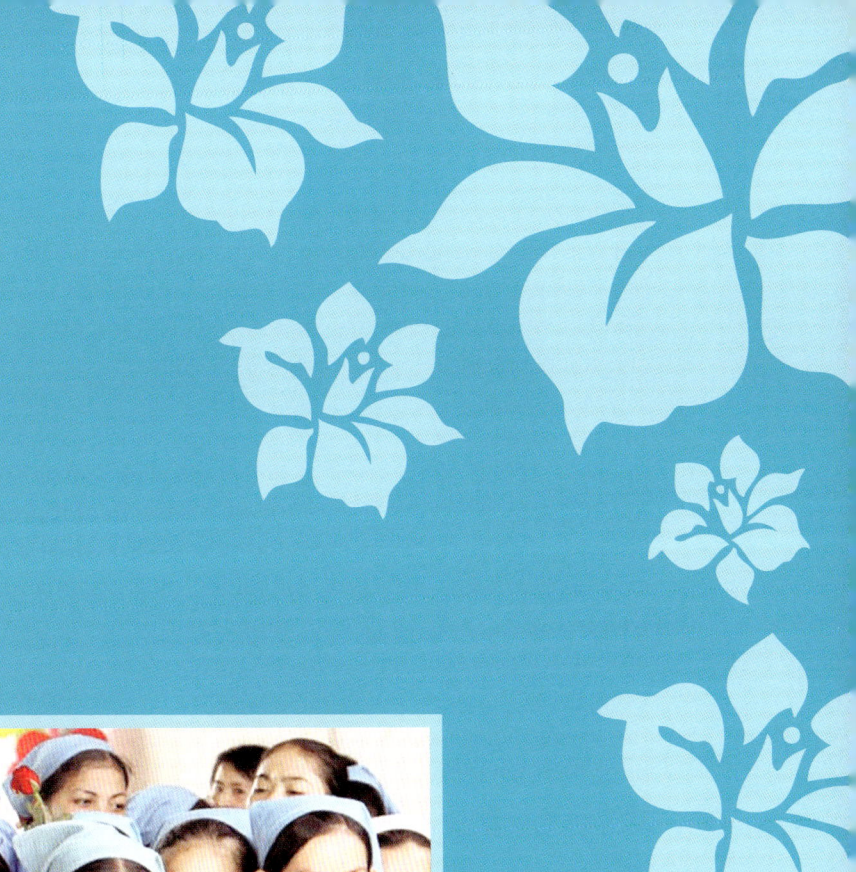
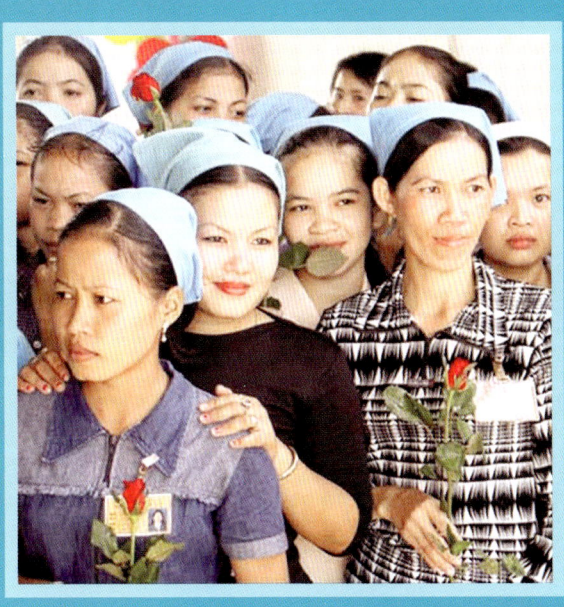

Section I : Background, objectives and methodology

Background

The global prevalence of anaemia is estimated to be 30.2% in non-pregnant women, rising to 41.8% during pregnancy[3]. Iron deficiency (ID) accounts for the majority of anaemia in most settings and affects two or more times the number of people who are anaemic. ID has important consequences that are independent of low haemoglobin levels.

Unfortunately, several approaches—in place for over half a century—have not been effective in preventing and controlling iron deficiency and anaemia, much less in increasing iron reserves in women of reproductive age (WRA). Improving iron and folate nutrition of WRA is known, not only to influence safe motherhood and birth outcomes, but also to enhance health and well-being by optimizing educational performance and increasing overall productivity. Urgent measures are required to improve the iron status of WRA using integrated approaches. Good health and nutrition, particularly the prevention of iron deficiency in WRA and the building of iron reserves prior to pregnancy, needs to be accorded a high priority in the development agenda at international, national and subnational levels.

The most desirable approaches to improving iron status are food-based:

1. dietary modification (increasing iron-rich foods and reducing absorption inhibitors);
2. bio-fortification to increase the iron content of staple crops; and
3. food fortification.

However, these are long-term solutions. In the short and medium terms, weekly iron folic acid supplementation (WIFS) programmes for populations at risk can make an important contribution to accelerating the achievement of the Millennium Development Goals (MDG) of improving child survival, maternal health and universal elementary education. WIFS for WRA, including adolescent girls, has been proven to be effective in several efficacy trials in Asia, the Pacific and Latin America. However, application of the findings to large-scale WIFS programmes for WRA is not well known.

Taking this into consideration, a WHO Global Consultation on Weekly Iron and Folic Acid Supplementation (WIFS) for Preventing Anaemia in Women of Reproductive Age (WRA) was held at the WHO Regional Office for the Western Pacific, in Manila, the Philippines, on 25-27 April 2007. The objectives of the consultation were:

1. to review the evidence for the efficacy, safety and feasibility of WIFS for preventing anaemia and improving the iron and folate status of women, before, during and after pregnancy;
2. to specify the conditions under which this approach could be successfully implemented in WRA at national or regional levels;

> **Improving iron and folate nutrition of WRA is known, not only to influence safe motherhood and birth outcomes, but also to enhance health and well-being by optimizing educational performance and increasing overall productivity.**

> **A successful WIFS programme can improve:**
> - maternal health;
> - foetal health;
> - child survival;
> - work productivity; and
> - school performance.

---

3   See Ref 2.

3. to decide on possible recommendations and guidelines to apply this approach on a large scale in order to increase the effectiveness of programmes to prevent and control anaemia and iron deficiency; and

4. to identify and prioritize knowledge gaps for which additional research is needed.

The scope for integrating WIFS programmes into other public health interventions and development programmes, such as education and women's development, to improve iron status and reduce the prevalence of anaemia was emphasized. In that context, it was identified that one of the required research areas was analysis of successful WIFS programmes to identify critical elements for taking to scale, including determinants of compliance with WIFS and ways to increase compliance. As a follow-up to the consultation, a study was launched in January 2008 with the following objectives and methodology.

Objectives of the study

1. To identify large-scale global WIFS programmes for WRA.
2. To review and present information on WIFS programmes in the form of case studies.
3. To undertake an analysis of case studies to identify the processes used for effective implementation of the various WIFS programmes.
4. To identify the best programme implementation practices, including ways to increase compliance.

Methodology

In order to achieve the objectives of the study, the first step was identification of large-scale WIFS programmes for WRA with the following criteria:

- WIFS programmes with a focus, not on efficacy trials, but on large-scale implementation to improve iron status and control iron deficiency and anaemia.
- A clearly defined geographical area.
- Availability of published or unpublished reports that include information on the implementation process.
- A representation of countries from across the continents.

The existing global published and unpublished literature and programme documents on WIFS in WRA were reviewed. The WRA group included adolescent girls aged 10-19 years and women up to the age of 49 years. In order to adhere to the above criteria, published efficacy studies or research findings of small-scale projects with valuable information on impact or approaches were excluded. Similarly, a number of published studies on using WIFS for young or primary-school children were also not included in the study.

To understand the process adequately and to convert the information into a case-study format with the required details, a standard template was developed (Annex 1). The standard template was completed with the information obtained from the synthesis of published papers in scientific journals as well as programme evaluation reports. However, as the data available from those sources were often found to be inadequate, reports, in the form of field visit and programme progress reports, were also obtained and reviewed. Additionally, information gaps were filled in by contacting the implementers and nodal contact people for the programmes. Information was analysed and documented in the form of case studies and was further synthesised to summarize the lessons learnt in planning and implementing WIFS programmes.

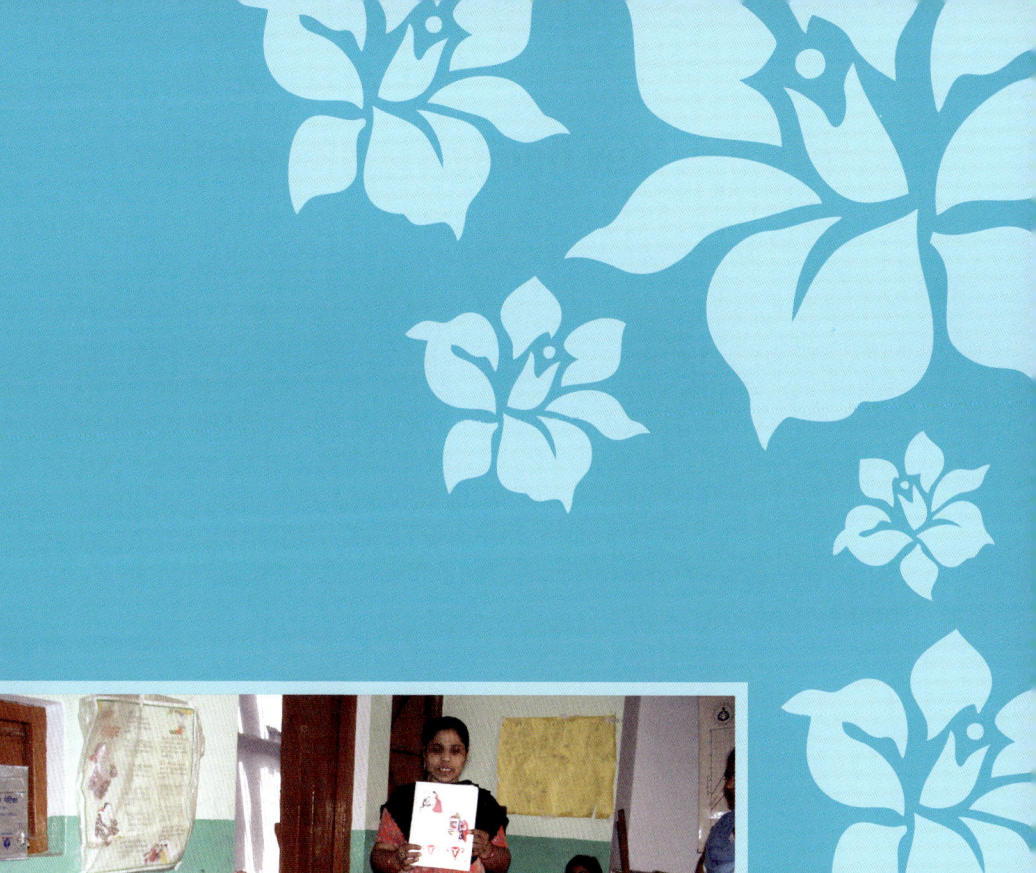

Section II : Global WIFS programmes for WRA — an analysis

- Section II A: Key findings and observations
- Section II B: Best programme practices

Section II A: Key findings and observations

1. WIFS programmes reviewed — an overview

A total of 19 WIFS programmes targeting WRA, including 13 Indian programmes, were identified during the review process. However, only four Indian programmes fitted the selection criteria. A total of 10 large-scale programmes across six countries were finally identified and reviewed. Those WIFS programmes were implemented over the period from 1998 to 2008, and covered over 2.5 million WRA. Six of the 10 programmes were from two countries, but with distinct strategy and implementation processes, two from Viet Nam and four from India. The other four programmes were from Cambodia, Egypt, the Lao People's Democratic Republic and the Philippines (Table 1).

2. Strategies utilized in WIFS programmes

All 10 programmes, except the programme in Yen Bai Province in Viet Nam, targeted adolescent girls in school, while five programmes also targeted WRA in communities or factories (Table 1). All four Indian programmes reached girls in and out of school. The central intervention strategy was either:

- provision of iron-folic acid supplements (IFA) free of cost to WRA, complemented by an appropriate communication strategy; or
- selling of IFA tablets to WRA with a strong demand created for WIFS through a social marketing approach (Table 1).

The latter included programmes in Cambodia, the Philippines and Hai Duong Province in Viet Nam. WRA in the community were reached in three programmes: Cambodia, the Lao People's Democratic Republic and Yen Bai Province (Viet Nam), the latter two providing WIFS free of cost to WRA in community settings.

Intensive social marketing strategies, focusing on the "four Ps" of marketing (product, price, place and promotion), were used by Cambodia, the Lao People's Democratic Republic, the Philippines and Hai Duong Province in Viet Nam. Across all 10 programmes, a fixed "WIFS Day" or "Iron Day" strategy was used to aid programme management and improve compliance (Table 1). The traditional approach of accessing non-pregnant WRA and adolescent girls through health clinics was found to be unfeasible. Therefore, WIFS were introduced through such institutions as schools or factories, or by mobilizing women's unions or community groups.

Successful strategies ensured an uninterrupted supply of good quality IFA, which was accessible at an affordable cost.

3. Intervention packages

Two interventions were found to be common across all 10 programmes: weekly iron-folic supplementation and promotion of dietary intake of iron-rich food. The latter was included as part of nutrition education or family-life education. In six of the 10 programmes, biannual administration of deworming was included in the intervention package (Table 1). The cost of the programme/WRA/year varied from

> **Two interventions were common across all 10 programmes: weekly iron-folic supplementation and promotion of dietary intake of iron-rich food.**

US$0.15 to US$5/day. The cost was significantly higher in programmes that sold tablets and used intensive, social marketing support materials and mass-media channels, such as television and print advertising. The WIFS programmes that were up-scaled in four of the six countries were based on the free supply of WIFS to WRA (Table 1).

Composition, packaging and cost of IFA supplements

As presented in Table 1, the elemental iron content in the IFA supplement for all the WIFS programmes, except the Indian programmes, was 60 mg, in the form of ferrous sulphate. In India, tablets contained 100 mg of elemental iron in the form of ferrous sulphate. The folic acid content in the IFA supplements varied widely, the lowest being 0.3 mg and the highest 3.5 mg per tablet. No rationale was presented for the variation in composition of the supplement; generally, however, the lower doses of folic acid corresponded to those found in daily iron/folic acid supplements, which were used in some projects as weekly supplements, while the higher dose (3.5 mg) was used in Cambodia, the Lao People's Democratic Republic, the Philippines and Viet Nam based on previous efficacy studies aimed at providing sufficient folic acid supplementation for one week.

Tablets were mostly supplied in blister packs of 4, 5, 10 or 30. The price of the annual IFA supplement of 52 tablets varied from a very low price of US$0.12 to a high price of US$3.64 (Table 1). The price of the supplement was much higher in those countries where social marketing strategies were used, due to the additional cost of packaging and promotional materials. The profit margin built into the cost of the supplement also contributed to the higher price. In these programmes, the price of the product was fixed in consultation with WRA in the community, since it was essential that WRA could access supplements at an affordable price (Table 1).

Demand creation

Education and social marketing were integral parts of all 10 programmes and were used to ensure a demand for IFA supplements and convince the target population to consume the product regularly. Education on WIFS was always accompanied by information to influence dietary behaviour and use of iron-rich foods. For adolescent girls, WIFS education was part of family-life education in two of the four Indian programmes, which helped in sustaining the interest of WRA. In school, the use of non-formal education modules was observed to be effective.

The information and education activities were either traditional or well planned social marketing strategies. The education component was more intensive and systematic in five programmes (Cambodia, Egypt, the Lao People's Democratic Republic, the Philippines and Hai Duong Province in Viet Nam), where the communication strategies and action plans were based on findings from formative research. Health and nutrition education improved acceptance of WIFS and compliance. While the use of social marketing was effective, it significantly increased the cost of programmes, as evidenced by project cost per WRA (Table 1). The social marketing approach was also more complex, since it focused on motivating target groups to adapt their behaviour rather than just the provision of supplements and consumption. In some social marketing programmes, funds generated from the sale of WIFS were used for programme implementation, which had the advantage of increasing programme sustainability.

Capacity-building

The importance of building the capacity of teachers, health workers and community leaders was noted across the projects. In most WIFS programmes, the health sector was in charge of training due to the inclusion of technical information on ID, such as causes and prevention. In all the programmes, training included information on dietary sources of iron and dietary inhibitors of iron absorption. Information on side-effects and the importance of consuming WIFS was adequately emphasized. However, despite the fact that community discussion on the benefits of WIFS was found to play a critical role in improving compliance, the benefits of WIFS that would be experienced by WRA in day-to-day activities was only adequately addressed in a few programmes. In most programmes, training content included components on skill-building for logistics management, counselling, conducting group education sessions, organization of social mobilization activities and monitoring.

Monitoring, supervision and compliance

Standard individual monitoring forms or monitoring registers in institutions, such as schools and factories, were effective in monitoring supply and consumption. In some of the WIFS programmes, easy-to-use cards for individuals were also effective, with demonstrated benefits in compliance. However, practical programme constraints were reported when such a system of individual monitoring cards was put in operation on a very large scale. Supervision during consumption of WIFS proved unfeasible in large-scale programmes. In programmes based on the sale of WIFS to WRA, no supervision component was included, but monitoring of sales was built in. Similarly, supervision during consumption was not feasible in many programmes because WRA were advised, in order to reduce side-effects, to consume IFA supplements on a full stomach at night, prior to going to bed. Despite a lack of supervision, however, a number of programmes such as those in Cambodia, the Lao People's Democratic Republic, the Philippines, and Uttar Pradesh and Bihar in India reported a high compliance rate for WIFS (Table 2). This may be attributed to the positive impact of the monitoring of supply and consumption of IFA supplements, built into the programme design. Establishing an effective monitoring mechanism, regular counselling and educating WRA regarding the impact of WIFS on health and beauty appeared to be far more critical than the supervision of WIFS consumption in securing compliance. This conclusion is well supported by findings from a comparison study of supervised and non-supervised WIFS consumption from a programme in Uttar Pradesh, India, which reported no difference in the percentage anaemia reduction in an adolescent girls group who consumed WIFS under supervision compared with those who did not.

Despite the fact that community discussion on the benefits of WIFS was found to play a critical role in improving compliance, the benefits of WIFS that would be experienced by WRA in day-to-day activities was only adequately addressed in a few programmes.

Establishing an effective monitoring mechanism, regular counselling and educating WRA regarding the impact of WIFS on health and beauty appeared to be far more critical than the supervision of WIFS consumption in securing compliance.

Table 1: An overview of 10 selected WIFS programmes

Central strategy	WIFS programme (year)	Target population - Adolescent girls - School	Adolescent girls - Non-school	Community	WRAs[c] - Institution (other than school)	Composition - Elemental iron (mg)	Composition - Folic acid (mg)	WIFS - Fixed day	Intervention - Cost/year (52 weeks) (US $)	Supply source	Biannual deworming	Education and social mobilization (Nutrition, family-life education, social marketing)	Programme cost (US $) per WRA / year	WIFS scaled up[d]
IFA supplied free of cost to WRA	Bihar, India (2000)	x	x	-	-	100	0.5	Wednesday	0.12	UNICEF & State Government	x	x	0.32	x
	Bihar, India (2000)	x	x	-	-	100	0.5	Wednesday	0.12	UNICEF & State Government	-	x	0.15[f]	x
	Madhya Pradesh, India (2002)	x	x	-	-	100	0.5	Tuesday / Saturday	0.12	UNICEF & State Government	x	x	0.33	x
	Uttar Pradesh, India (2001)	x	x	-	-	100	0.5	Saturday	0.12	UNICEF & State Government	x	x	0.36	x
	Egypt[a] (1999)	x	-	-	-	60	0.3	Monday	Not stated[i]	Not stated	x[e]	x	0.36-0.50	x
	Lao People's Democratic Republic (2006)	x	-	x	-	60	3.5	Monday	Not stated	United Laboratories, Inc. (UNILAB)	x	x[h]	10-12[g]	~
	Yen Bai Province, Viet Nam (2006)	-	-	x	-	60	0.4	Locally decided day	0.40	NAPHACO (government)	x	x	Not presented	x
IFA purchased by WRA	Cambodia[b] (2001)	x	-	x	x (factory)	60	3.5	Saturday	130	UNILAB	x	x[h]	5[g]	x
	Philippines[b] (1998)	x	-	x	-	60	3.5	Tuesday	364	UNILAB	-	x[h]	5[g]	~
	Hai Duong Province, Viet Nam (1999)	x	-	x	-	60 / 60	3.5 / 0.4[j]	Locally decided day	104 / 39	UNILAB and government	-	x[h]	5[g]	x

a Adolescent boys were also included ~ scaling up under review
b Social marketing approach with WIFS purchased by WRA. The Lao People's Democratic Republic used the social marketing approach to creating demand, but provided WIFS free of cost.
c WRA or women of reproductive age includes adolescent girls.
d All scaled-up strategy is based on free supply of WIFS.
e Deworming is a separate national programme
f Low cost since no deworming and excludes cost of management.
g Cost estimated based on total project cost divided by the number of WRA covered (in the pilot phase).
h Social marketing approach used.
i In 2009, new formula was used with 120 mg ferrous fumerate and 0.3 mg Folic acid, costing US$ 0.26-0.31 for 52 tablets.
j In phase 2, the composition was changed as per government policy. Supply was also procured by the government.
~ Scaling up is part of government policy and/or in progress.

WIFS compliance was high, reported to be about 70% or above in all WIFS programmes except one (Table 2). The incidence of adverse side-effects reported was low, at 5.3% to 18.7%, and was not found to be a major programme constraint. Compliance improved significantly when information, education and communication (IEC) activities emphasized the benefits of WIFS rather than just the side-effects. The positive impact of WIFS on:

- improved concentration and school performance;
- improved energy output and reduced fatigue;
- enhanced skin glow and improved appearance; and
- regularization of menstruation.

was appealing and convincing, since the WRA experienced these benefits and associated the effects with regular consumption of WIFS. A system to share such benefits experienced by other WRA in institutions or community groups was encouraged and proved effective in promoting compliance.

Table 2: WIFS — Compliance and anaemia reduction prevalence rates

WIFS programme	Intervention period (months)	Compliance (%)	Anaemia prevalence (baseline) (%)	Reduction in anaemia prevalence (%)
Bihar, India	12	85-92.2	93.0	9.3
Gujarat, India	12	89-94	74.7	28.8
Madhya Pradesh, India	16	92	87.8	8.9
Uttar Pradesh, India	12	86-90	73.3	46.8
Egypt	6	92.2	30.0	20.0
Lao People's Democratic Republic	7	74.5	43.0	53.4
Yen Bai Province, Viet Nam	12	69	37.5	48.0
Cambodia	7	44-71	58.0	-
Philippines	12	95	33.3	-
Hai Duong Province, Viet Nam	9	54-92	45.6	56.8

Forgetfulness was noted to be an important factor in poor compliance (Table 3). A fixed "WIFS Day" strategy was used in each of the 10 programmes to address that issue, as well as to improve the overall management of the programme. The choice of days used as "WIFS day" or "Anaemia Day" varied in different situations.

For schools, the Egyptian programme considered Monday to be the most suitable WIFS day, since attendance of students was reported to be highest on that day and the scope of tracking a drop-out case within the week itself was considered most practical. The WIFS programme of Gujarat used Wednesday as the WIFS day since, in consultation with school authorities, it was found that this was the most common day for not observing any religious fast (Table 1). In the Philippines,

Tuesday was declared WIFS Day, since Wednesday was the fixed immunization day and therefore the most appropriate and practical day for undertaking follow-up monitoring by the health immunization team. In the case of Yen Bai Province in Viet Nam, no special day was designated as WIFS Day for the entire programme, but WRA were counselled to select a suitable day in the week for WIFS consumption.

Table 3: WIFS percentage compliance rate and factors responsible		
	India (adolescent girls, non-school)	Lao People's Democratic Republic (WRA)
WIFS routinely taken (%)	86.0	74.5
WIFS not taken (%)	14.0	25.5
• Forgetfulness	52.4	50.0
• Side-effects (vomiting, stomach ache, health problems)	28.6	5.8
• Onset of pregnancy		16.7
• Other	19.0	27.5

* Only 4% of total adolescent girls studied complained of adverse effects

In all programmes, except in the Lao People's Democratic Republic and the Philippines, active efforts were made to counsel WRA on how to reduce side-effects and increase compliance. WRA in most programmes were advised to consume WIFS prior to going to bed and to use safe water for swallowing. Tea and coffee drinking for swallowing tablets or soon after consumption of iron-folic acid supplements was actively discouraged. The finding that unpleasant side-effects decreased as time of usage of WIFS increased was also communicated to WRA to reduce the number of drop-outs and increase compliance.

Research shows that WIFS is an effective strategy, with a high compliance rate, for reducing the prevalence of anaemia in WRA.

4. Impact on anaemia prevalence

Reductions in anaemia prevalence rates were reported for eight of the 10 WIFS programmes, ranging from 8.9% to 56.8% over an intervention period of 6 to 16 months (Table 2). In the absence of any control group, it is not feasible to analyse the factors contributing to such a wide variation. However, it is interesting to note that, in programmes where anaemia prevalence at the start of the programme was over 85% (93.5% in Bihar, India, and 87.8 % in Madhya Pradesh, India), the overall reduction in anaemia prevalence was much lower and within the range of 8.7% to 9.8%. An analysis of data from Madhya Pradesh indicates that, in the first 16 months of intervention, there was a significant decrease in moderate anaemia cases and a shift towards mild anaemia. It is possible that a longer intervention with WIFS would result in shifting the mild cases of anaemia to a non-anaemic status. Moreover, other causative factors may be responsible for the reduced impact of WIFS. In Uttar Pradesh, the Lao People's Democratic Republic and Viet Nam, the reduction in anaemia prevalence achieved in 7 to 12 months was about 50% or greater.

5. Scaling up strategies

Seven out of eight of the scaled-up programmes were based on a free supply of supplements (Table 1), with political support and commitment facilitating the process. Integration with effective existing delivery systems in health, education and the private sector (e.g. factories, women's groups, schools, market networks and local shops), as well as community organizations, proved effective.

In India, the Anaemia Control Programme for Adolescents has been built into the school health programme of the National Rural Health Mission (NRHM) in many states of the country. This is because one third of adolescent girls in India begin childbearing at the young age of 19 years[4] and the significance of building pre-pregnancy iron stores through WIFS is well appreciated. The supplement is provided free of cost by the government health system.

In Egypt, with substantial political support, the WIFS programme has been taken to scale, with about 6 million adolescents being reached. In fact, Egypt is the only country where both adolescent boys and girls have been included as beneficiaries of the WIFS programme. The positive impact of WIFS has resulted in various countries, such as Cambodia, India, the Lao People's Democratic Republic, Panama, the Philippines and Viet Nam, recognising the importance of including a WIFS programme as part of their nutrition and health policies.

It is evident from the WIFS programmes analysed in this study that political support needs to be sought to ensure an uninterrupted supply of supplements and for effective implementation of WIFS. Developing the capacity of governments or building strong partnerships with private pharmaceutical sectors to produce quality supplements is therefore essential. Additionally, adequate funds need to be allocated by governments to finance multi-media advertising, including the use of mass media, in order to create a sustained demand for WIFS. The strategy adopted by a particular country needs to take into account the fact that WIFS is a long-term intervention and therefore effort must be made to make the programme commercially self-sustainable. A two-pronged approach should therefore be considered: free supply of WIFS along with intensive education for the lower socioeconomic WRA, and a policy for promoting the sale of WIFS to the remaining population using a social marketing approach.

It is evident from the WIFS programmes analysed in this study that political support needs to be sought to ensure an uninterrupted supply of supplements and for effective implementation of WIFS.

---

4   *National Family Health Survey (NFHS-3), 2005-06, Volume II.* Mumbai, International Institute for Population Sciences.

Section II B: Best programme practices

A total of 10 large-scale WIFS programmes for WRA were analysed to synthesize the best programme strategy and activities for improving iron and folate status and reducing anaemia prevalence in WRA. The information presented in this section is intended to serve as a planning and implementation guide for policy-makers, programme managers and planners of WIFS programmes.

1. Assessing iron deficiency and anaemia problems

> It is essential to create a database on the prevalence of anaemia and ID in WRA prior to considering the introduction of WIFS as a public health measure in a region. Information on causative factors of ID is important in deciding the most effective action needed to improve iron nutrition among WRA.

It is well documented that ID is the single most common cause of anaemia in pregnant women, as well as the WRA group, which includes adolescent girls aged 10-19 years who have attained menarche. According to international criteria, ID and IDA is a severe public health problem in a region when the prevalence of anaemia is 40% or above. It is a moderate public health problem if anaemia prevalence is between 20%-39%[5]. Haemoglobin cut-off values for defining anaemia in various population groups and for assessing anaemia prevalence are presented in Table 4. Once IDA is established as a public health problem, building pre-pregnancy iron stores and preventing anaemia in WRA is essential. Surveys and secondary information need to be reviewed in order to understand the factors contributing to ID and to work out an implementation plan to prevent and control anaemia in WRA.

Table 4: Haemoglobin and haematocrit cut-offs used to define anaemia in people living at sea level

Age or sex group	Haemoglobin level (g/dl)	Haematocrit below (%)
Children 6 months to 4 years	11.0	33
Children 5 -11 years	11.5	34
Children 12 -14 years	12.0	36
Non-pregnant women	12.0	36
Pregnant women	11.0	33
Men	13.0	39

Source: *Iron deficiency anaemia: assessment, prevention, and control. A guide for programme managers.* Geneva, World Health Organization, 2001 (WHO/NHD/01.3).

---

5 *Preventing ID in women and children: Technical consensus on key issues.* A UNICEF/UNU/WHO/MI technical workshop, 7-9 October 1998.

2. Revisiting the anaemia control programme strategies in countries

> In countries where IDA is a public health problem, it is vital to move beyond strengthening anaemia control programmes that address only pregnant women. In developing countries, high priority must be accorded to building iron nutrition prior to pregnancy, as this is critical for the health of WRA and reduces risk during pregnancy. It is essential to involve various stakeholders, including multiprogramme and private sector representatives, particularly from the pharmaceutical industry, in formulating a successful WIFS implementation strategy.

The problem of ID and anaemia should be viewed, not only as a serious public health problem during pregnancy, but also as a serious health problem in WRA. Existing anaemia prevention and management policies therefore need to be reviewed to consider the inclusion of preventive measures such as WIFS for WRA in the public health policy of the country. Reviews of programmes reveal that WIFS is a practical strategy for preventing anaemia in non-pregnant WRA and results in a number of benefits, such as:

- reducing tiredness and improving sleep patterns;
- increasing appetite;
- increasing energy levels and working capacity;
- improving learning ability and school performance;
- improving immune function;
- regularizing menstruation and improving iron stores in non-pregnant women; and
- building pre-pregnancy iron stores.

The recommendations of the *WHO Global Consultation and the WHO position statement on WIFS for WRA* (Annex 2), combined with examples of successful WIFS case studies (Section III) could form the basis for national consultations towards revisiting the programme strategy for anaemia control. To formulate such a strategy, it is important that national consultations are not confined to the health and nutrition sectors of government, but involve wider participation, including representatives from: departments of education; women's development; rural development; youth development; mass communication; and sections of the private sector that primarily have a female workforce, such as garment factories and tea estates; pharmaceutical groups; advertising agencies; and social marketing agencies.

3. Advocacy and formulation of policy

In order to place improvement of iron nutrition and reduction of anaemia high on the political agenda, advocacy needs to emphasize the economic and health benefits of WIFS for WRA and the cost-effectiveness of this intervention. Developing policies regarding the prevention of ID and anaemia in WRA is essential in securing resources and funding, establishing successful programme strategies and legitimizing and sustaining implementation of WIFS programmes. A high-profile launch is useful in mobilizing political support.

It is crucial to inform policy-makers about the serious implications of ID and anaemia for school performance, pregnancy outcome and productivity. The important economic losses to countries and families as a result of ID and the corresponding gains achieved by preventing such deficiency need to be appreciated. Equally important is the need to inform all involved of the benefits of WIFS and the effects of such interventions on MDG progress. Table 5 highlights the relationship between anaemia control in WRA and the MDGs. Such information supports WIFS programme advocacy and facilitates decisions by policy-makers and planners to include WIFS programmes as part of measures to improve the health of WRA and improve iron status.

Policy-makers need to be made aware of the low cost of WIFS interventions compared with the high cost of ID and anaemia for national health, productivity and the economy. Case studies from three large-scale programmes in India and Egypt indicate that the annual cost of WIFS programmes for adolescent girls can be as low as US$0.15 to US$0.36 per recipient. IFA supplements make up only about one third of that total cost. Moreover, cost-analysis data from the Uttar Pradesh WIFS programme reveal that the total project cost per WRA is reduced significantly when programmes are taken to scale and cover a larger number of WRA. Sharing such information with policy-makers will aid in securing resources to address the serious public health issues caused by ID and anaemia, particularly in adolescent girls and pre-pregnant women.

Table 5: ID and IDA prevention in WRA through WIFS helps to achieve the MDGs

MDGs	Impact of IDA prevention
MDG # 1 Eradicate extreme poverty and hunger	• Increases the body's capacity to do work (for every 10% increase in HB — 15% increase in physical work). • Reduces low birth weight. • Reduces undernutrition in children under five years.
MDG # 2 Achieve universal primary education	• Reduces the frequency and severity of infections / morbidity and mortality. • Increases school attendance, retention, learning capacity and school achievement.
MDG # 3 Promote gender equality and empower women	• Reduces anaemia in girls — often more severe than in boys. Lack of iron adversely influences school attendance and achievement. • Reduces gender disparity.
MDG # 4 Reduce child mortality	• Reduces serious consequences on child health, including low birth-weight and stillbirth. • Reduces child mortality.
MDG # 5 Improve maternal health	• Reduces maternal anaemia. • Reduces the maternal mortality ratio (MMR) (20% of maternal deaths are directly attributed to anaemia).

Source: Cavalli-Sforza T, *et al*. Weekly iron folic acid supplementation of women of reproductive age: impact overview, lessons learned, expansion plans, and contributions toward achievement of the Millennium Development Goals. *Nutrition reviews*, December 2005; 63(12): S152-S158.

With a policy of WIFS for WRA in place, programme interventions are legitimized and this facilitates implementation. Establishing policies is essential for commitment to the programme and also for resource allocation, which helps in overcoming important political, programme, social and structural barriers. These issues are well reflected in the evolution of WIFS programmes in India and Egypt. In India, the recommendations of the National Consultation on Anaemia Control, held in 1997,[6] stated:

> *'Adolescent girls on attaining menarche should consume one IFA tablet containing 100mg elemental iron and 500 mcg folic acid once a week. This should be accompanied by appropriate dietary counselling. Considering the large size of the adolescent population as well as the financial and operational constraints, it is recommended that district-level pilot projects should be undertaken. The total duration of a weekly dose of iron supplements, its cost-effectiveness and operational feasibility should be examined.'*

This recommendation was followed by a launch of district- and state-level demonstration projects in many parts of India and finally by the inclusion of WIFS for adolescent girls in the State Implementation Plans of selected states under the National Rural Health Mission, Ministry of Health and Family Welfare.[7] Experience reveals that policy formulation, combined with a high-profile programme launch, facilitates in gaining political support during the implementation phase.

4. Target population and strategy for accessing IFA supplements

Anaemia programmes for WRA in developing countries include targeting adolescent girls both in and out of school, as well as WRA who are in communities or are part of the workforce. WIFS programmes ideally need to target WRA across all socioeconomic groups, since anaemia prevalence is often high irrespective of economic conditions. In order for all WRA to have access to WIFS, a strategy of providing free WIFS for economically disadvantaged WRA should be combined with promoting the purchase of WIFS, at a reasonable price, for women with a higher socioeconomic status, using a social marketing approach.

Distinct strategies should be used in designing WIFS programmes for four primary sections of the WRA population: adolescent girls in schools, adolescent girls out of school, women in factories or other workplaces or institutions, and women in communities. Non-pregnant WRA are a section of the population that is not routinely reached through the health sector. An effective way of reaching such women is by involving non-health sector partners and establishing links with various ongoing development programmes, as well as building on institutional or non-formal networks of WRA. Effective strategies for contacting and working

---

6 National Consultation on Control of Nutritional Anaemia in India, Nirman Bhavan, New Delhi, 16-17 October 1997, Ministry of Health and Family Welfare.

7 See Ref 5.

with WRA in WIFS programmes include reaching adolescent girls in schools, using a school-to-community approach, and selecting and training community volunteers, women union leaders, teachers and frontline workers in health and other development programmes dealing with WRA.

It is estimated that almost one third of adolescent girls in developing countries are married[8] and conceive within a year of marriage. Within the WRA group, designing and implementing WIFS programmes for adolescent girls has therefore been accorded a high= priority because of the need to build pre-pregnancy iron stores and prevent the serious complications of ID during pregnancy. Moreover, reaching this section of the WRA population is a good start in addressing anaemia in WRA, since females at this age are more responsive and motivated to take action when mobilized in school or community groups. Additionally, it is envisaged that establishing a habit of regularly consuming WIFS in adolescence will help build a habit of consuming IFA supplements in adulthood and will also improve compliance during pregnancy.

The senior school education sector, with or without involvement of the health sector, has been clearly shown to be the most effective channel for reaching adolescent girls in school in all four WIFS programmes in India and in other countries, such as Cambodia, Egypt and the Lao People's Democratic Republic. Experiences from developing countries demonstrate that the success of scaled-up programmes is also due to schoolgirls reaching out to disadvantaged girls who are not in school in a "girl-to-girl" or "girl-to-community" approach. This dimension of WIFS programmes for adolescent girls in schools adds further value to school-based WIFS programmes. A successfully implemented girl-to-girl approach involves forming a club or core group of 15-20 schoolgirls who are trained to be "nodal girls". Each nodal girl is assigned the responsibility of reaching a minimum of one to three adolescent girls who are not in school. The responsibility of regularly supplying IFA supplements, counselling on the benefits of regular weekly use of supplements, managing any side-effects reported and monitoring consumption by out-of-school girls have all been successfully carried out by schoolgirls who are trained and assigned those tasks. In fact, the Uttar Pradesh WIFS programme clearly indicates that girls assigned such responsibilities take pride in their tasks and are motivated by the fact that schoolteachers and the community recognize their contribution and view them as having special leadership qualities.

The components and strategies used in a WIFS programme are governed by the central decision on whether IFA supplements will be provided free of cost to WRA. Consumption of WIFS is expected to continue throughout the reproductive life cycle, until other ways of ensuring adequate iron and folic acid status in the population are achieved through dietary improvement. The policy of free distribution of WIFS to WRA is therefore an effective short-term strategy and has been the policy choice of developing countries, such as Cambodia, Egypt, India and Viet Nam, that have scaled up their programmes. As reported by the WIFS programme in Yen Bai Province in Viet Nam, provision of free IFA ensures equitable distribution and higher participation of poorer, more disadvantaged women, especially ethnic minorities. Since ID and anaemia in WRA is prevalent

---

8   See Ref 5.

across socioeconomic situations, a two-pronged strategy is needed, comprising free distribution of supplements to a defined low socioeconomic population and social marketing of the supplements at a reasonable cost to those WRA who can afford them. This, along with measures to promote the consumption of foods rich in iron, would provide a sustainable solution to improving iron status.

5. Composition, presentation and supply of IFA supplements

Documented case studies demonstrate that the specifications of IFA supplements with reference to composition, colour (red), size, shape (round or elliptical), coating of tablets, presentation details (such as packaging, nomenclature, attractiveness of illustration or labelling and information printed on benefits), and having a designated "WIFS Day/Iron Day", contribute significantly to the success of a WRA programme. Attractive blister packaging (4, 5 or 10 tablets per blister) enhances the value of the product. In the absence of availability of a distinct packaged product for weekly consumption by WRA, IFA tablets used daily during pregnancy could be successfully used for weekly consumption by WRA. For a WIFS programme to be successful, it is essential that an uninterrupted supply of good quality IFA supplements, at a low cost, is ensured through partnership with the private sector.

The 10 WIFS programmes reviewed indicate two levels of elemental iron in the IFA supplements used—60mg and 100mg—in the form of ferrous sulphate. The folic acid content of the supplements used varied widely, from 0.3mg to 3.5mg. It is evident from the case studies that, in situations where no special supplements are produced for WRA, IFA supplements designed for daily use during pregnancy can be successfully used as a weekly supplement for non-pregnant WRA. However, based on the research findings reviewed at the WHO Global Consultation on Weekly Iron and Folic Acid Supplementation for Preventing Anaemia in Women of Reproductive Age, held in Manila, Philippines, in 2007, IFA tablets for once-a-week consumption by WRA are recommended to contain a minimum of 60mg of elemental iron and a much higher level of folic acid of 2.8 mg per tablet. The increase is recommended to build proper folic acid storage at the pre-pregnancy stage to prevent neural-tube defects in newborn infants. (Annex 2). Although, for effective programme management, it is desirable to promote the use of an IFA supplement that is specifically designed and produced for WRA, the Indian programmes demonstrate that logistical management of IFA supplements, even when identical to the supply used for pregnant mothers, is feasible as well as safe and effective for non-pregnant women.

It is evident from the case studies that the colour and shape of IFA tablets are important factors in promoting their consumption. Red or pink IFA tablets are reportedly well accepted and are often associated with "strengthening the blood". Coating tablets with colour film also helps increase their stability and shelf life in different storage conditions and reduces the side-effects of nausea and vomiting, which are caused by gastric irritation. Sugar-coating tablets improves their taste, but should not be encouraged since it increases the chances of the IFA tablets being mistaken for sweets and swallowed by children, with grave, and in some cases fatal consequences (depending on the age of the child and number of tablets ingested). Small, elliptical tablets are reported to be well accepted and easy to swallow. Moreover, tablets with a distinct design and colour are beneficial so that they are not mistaken for contraceptives or sweets.

The experiences of various countries indicate that packaging IFA tablets attractively, not only increases the value of the product, but also contributes to a positive image and helps sustain interest and demand. Moreover, appropriate packaging contributes to ease of storage and monitoring. The number of tablets to be packaged in one pack or blister strip depends on what users can afford and the frequency of contact the delivery system has with WRA. It has been demonstrated that blister packs containing at least one month's supply of four tablets in a strip is practical for public health service providers and for marketing purposes. A blister pack of four or 10 WIFS tablets was reported to be acceptable to WRA who purchased WIFS in Cambodia, the Philippines and Hai Duong Province in Viet Nam. In the WIFS programme in Yen Bai Province in Viet Nam, however, blister packs were designed as tear-off strips of five tablets, which was practical for free distribution. In all four India-based WIFS programmes, tablets were supplied free of cost in lots of four to five tablets or 10 tablets. The WIFS blisters of 4-10 tablets were cut from blister-pack sheets of 30 tablets that were used for supplying a minimum of 90 IFA supplement tablets during the three antenatal visits with pregnant mothers. This system is practical, since no special tablets need to be produced or packed for the weekly supplies for non-pregnant women and adolescent girls.

It is evident that each country needs to review and agree on the form and composition of supplements for its WIFS programme for WRA. In cases where IFA supplements are provided free of cost by the Government or another channel, the number of tablets to be included in each blister pack will be governed by the frequency of contact between providers and recipients, as well as the convenience of monitoring supply and consumption. In cases where WIFS are purchased, a market study should be carried out to determine the optimum number of tablets and the price that WRA are willing and able to pay for them, both in the short term and over several years.

The quality and attractiveness of packaging add to the cost of IFA supplements. In India, the cost to the Government of purchasing a mass supply of IFA supplements is only about US$ 0.12 for a one-year supply of 52 IFA tablets, with each tablet containing 100 mg of elemental iron and 0.5 mg of folic acid. In the Philippines, WIFS supplements were not supplied free of cost but were sold in pharmacies at a much higher price of about US$ 0.14 for just one tablet. The supplements had a much higher folic acid content (3.5mg) than the Indian supplements and a lower iron content (60mg). Moreover, they were produced and supplied by a private pharmaceutical agency in attractive, colourful packs, with the objective of creating market demand.

In situations where WIFS for WRA are part of a government-managed public health programme, the packaging cost needs to be reduced to a minimum. In cases where the central strategy is for WRA to purchase WIFS, supply and packaging design should be such that supplements are easily affordable but still attractive enough to enhance compliance. The case studies demonstrate that it is very useful to have information regarding the best time to take the tablets, the benefits of WIFS and the designated WIFS day printed on cartons or packages of IFA supplements. A product name and positive illustration on packs also increases acceptance, demand and purchase. A distinct, attractive logo highlighting the association of IFA supplements with health and beauty, further increases the value of the supplement for WRA and helps to achieve a shift from viewing WIFS as a medicine to a long-term strategy for protection of health and beauty.

The conclusions and recommendations of the 2007 WHO Global Consultation on WIFS, featuring criteria for ensuring the quality of iron and folic acid supplement tablets, are reported in Annex 3. An external quality monitoring mechanism is useful and needs to be put in place for periodic checking of the quality of IFA supplements. Establishing such a system will ensure that the approved standards of composition and quality are maintained. Additionally, countries should aim to develop the capacity of local pharmaceutical companies to produce supplements of accepted quality, with the right composition and appropriate packaging and cost.

6. Procurement and delivery of IFA supplements

It is critical to ensure the availability of resources and the appropriate management of supplies, including correctly estimating requirements, so that there is an adequate supply of IFA supplements for the WIFS programme. Supply channels, based on the country's agreed strategy, need to be clearly defined so that supply is streamlined. Also, as IFA supplements need to be made available and accessible to WRA of various ages, in a wide range of situations, dependency on a single delivery system is not advisable. Dovetailing WIFS programmes with other available infrastructures and networks, particularly the education sector, is feasible, sustainable and low-cost. Marketing supplements using social marketing strategies is effective when WIFS are readily available for purchase at an affordable price through various community groups, NGOs and other institutional set-ups.

Establishing a mechanism for streamlining an uninterrupted supply of IFA tablets, whether they are distributed free of cost or through a social marketing strategy, is critical for ensuring a regular supply on a long-term basis. Supply of WIFS to nodal government departments, if the Government is in partnership with the private system, improves the sustainability of WIFS programmes. Pilot testing and establishing a suitable supply system is essential prior to scaling up a WIFS programme.

The annual supply requirement for WRA can be estimated by multiplying 52 tablets/person/year by the estimated number of WRA recipients, with an additional 20% for buffer stock. Taking into consideration the resources and storage facilities available, the entire annual supply of IFA could be procured at one time to reduce cost, since IFA supplements have a good shelf life. Channels for supply of IFA supplements, from production to procurement to service providers to consumers, will depend entirely on whether the IFA tablets are distributed free of charge or marketed to WRA. Allocating resources and defining the roles and responsibilities of government sectors, the private pharmaceutical industry and donors will ensure an adequate and consistent supply. An external system could be established by the Government, in partnership with private industry, if required, for periodic checking of the quality and logistical management of IFA supplements.

It is evident from the experiences of the WIFS programmes in various countries that it is not practical or cost-effective to be dependent on a single delivery channel, such as health, to optimize coverage of the target population. Dovetailing WIFS programmes with other available infrastructures and networks is feasible, sustainable and cost-effective. Adolescent girls in schools are easily reached by establishing a link with the middle- and secondary-school system. Teachers can be well accepted by schoolgirls as distributors and monitors of IFA supplements. For example, during the one-month Ramadan period in Egypt, the WIFS programme demonstrated that the supplements continued to be used at home by students providing the school supplied the WIFS and teachers directed students to consume the supplements about two hours after breaking their fast with a meal.

In situations where free supply of WIFS to WRA is implemented as a part of a public health programme, teachers, female leaders and leaders of religious institutions have been accepted by the community as credible and effective distributors. It has been estimated in the WIFS programme in Egypt that tablet distribution by a teacher to about 45 students in a class requires about 10-15 minutes. For effective distribution of WIFS, it is crucial that the location and frequency of distribution is specified and widely disseminated to WRA and the community. The availability of drinking water must also be ensured at distribution points in institutional or community set-ups.

> **Purchase of WIFS through a social marketing approach, rather than free supply, can be a sustainable solution, since WRA need to consume WIFS throughout their entire reproductive lives, unless iron-rich food or iron/folic-acid-fortified food is readily available to the population.**

In situations where WRA can afford to buy IFA supplements, social marketing has been used successfully as a strategy for reaching non-pregnant WRA. In Cambodia, for example, responses to buying IFA supplements were better in higher socioeconomic groups compared with lower ones. A social marketing strategy is of particular significance for non-pregnant, non-adolescent women of higher socioeconomic groups who are also anaemic but are not reached by the public health system. Moreover, purchase of WIFS through a social marketing approach, rather than free supply, is a sustainable solution, since WRA need to consume WIFS throughout their entire reproductive lives, unless iron-rich food or iron/folic-acid-fortified food is readily available to the population.

The planning and implementation of an effective social marketing programme has demonstrated positive results in terms of demand creation, sustaining satisfactory sales and high compliance. A successful social marketing strategy requires a quality IFA supplement product being available at the correct price and place. Ensuring the availability of and access to IFA supplements at an affordable price in traditional drug stores and local village or urban shops encourages WRA to buy the supplements as over-the-counter products. Additionally, IFA supplements can be made readily available and accessible through various groups, including: NGOs, networks of community volunteers, community development programmes, self-help groups, micro-credit groups of women, marriage registration systems, centres for family planning, centres for family welfare, centres for women's development and youth programmes, as well as through networking with organized and non-organized WRA groups employed in factories and other workplaces.

The role of private partnership with the pharmaceutical sector is of special significance since it has demonstrably contributed, not only to ensuring a regular supply of supplements, but also to promoting regular use of WIFS through appropriate marketing strategies based on the findings of community-specific market research. However, as indicated by the Philippines' WIFS programme, it is essential that government policy on WIFS for WRA contains a statement on the role of the private sector in preventing anaemia in order to sustain the interest and long-term involvement of the private pharmaceutical industry.

7. Communication strategy to create demand and improve coverage and compliance

Complementing the regular supply of IFA supplements with an effective communication strategy is a critical factor in the success of WIFS programmes, and formative research is useful in the development of such strategies. Sharing the benefits of WIFS experienced by WRA in peer-group discussions has been demonstrated to be a very effective communication strategy, while disseminating information on the day designated as "WIFS Day" and promoting consumption of WIFS on this day facilitates increased compliance. A social marketing approach, while it can be expensive, has long-term benefits and could be used in WIFS programmes to motivate target groups and influence the adoption of positive purchasing and consumption behaviour. Social mobilization actions, such as high-profile launches, mass media broadcasts, and community-based activities like rallies, debates, folk songs, etc., are critical in creating a supportive community environment.

One of the most important components of a WIFS programme is the communication strategy, which should have the following three main objectives:

1. To grant high priority to the WIFS programme.
2. To create demand for iron-folic acid tablets.
3. To motivate the target population to regularly consume the supplements.

In developing an effective communication strategy, including social mobilization and social marketing, an essential first step is to conduct formative research on the current knowledge, attitudes and practices related to iron and folic acid deficiency, anaemia and its prevention. Such research needs to be conducted among all WRA, including adolescent girls both in and out of school, non-adolescent and newly married women, pregnant and lactating women, influential members of the community, youth and female leaders, and university students. Additionally, it is advantageous to include other stakeholders in the study, such as policy-makers, programme managers, providers of health services and education, women's development institutions, women's workplace and community leaders, and pharmaceutical managers.

The research should aim to seek information regarding:

- dietary practices and sources of iron and folate;
- facilitating factors and barriers to acquiring IFA supplements for WRA;
- attitudes and practices related to regularly purchasing and taking IFA tablets;
- issues related to the supply of IFA supplements;
- views on optimal presentation of the product in terms of colour, shape, packaging and price;
- viable channels for distribution or purchase of IFA tablets; and
- acceptability of WIFS by front-line workers in the health and non-health sectors.

WIFS programmes in Cambodia, Egypt, the Lao People's Democratic Republic, the Philippines and Hai Duong Province in Viet Nam have demonstrated that comprehensive formative research can provide useful insights for appropriate positioning of the product, communication messages, logo design and standardization of the information to be printed on IFA packages. Moreover, research findings can also assist in the formulation of communication strategies, including the use of specific communication channels, such as interpersonal communications, multiple communication channels, mass media (TV and radio) and local community-based programmes (skits and health fairs, etc). The communication campaign and related support materials, as well as tools for counselling and for creating a supportive environment, should be based, as far as possible, on the results of formative research. Findings from the WIFS programme in Egypt also revealed that formative research can be useful in identifying innovative methods to motivate students and caregivers.

An analysis of the case studies revealed that IFA supplements should be positioned, not as a medicine to cure anaemia, but as a positive intervention, along with dietary measures, to improve iron status, prevent IDA and enhance the overall quality of life.

An analysis of the case studies revealed that IFA supplements should be positioned, not as a medicine to cure anaemia, but as a positive intervention, along with dietary measures, to improve iron status, prevent IDA and enhance the overall quality of life. The WIFS programme in the Philippines revealed that, in order to translate awareness of the significance of WIFS into the practice of regularly purchasing and consuming IFA supplements, it is vital that communication strategies encourage WRA to perceive WIFS as a measure for improving health and appearance, rather than as a therapeutic product. However, communication efforts still need to educate the community regarding common symptoms, such as dizziness, fatigue and paleness, which are often due to ID and can be prevented through the regular use of WIFS.

The focus of the communication action plan should be to sensitize all stakeholders at various levels — from health and education planners to service providers of WIFS — regarding the wide range of benefits of IFA. A comprehensive communication strategy should:

- address the relevant target groups;
- impact policy-makers, to encourage them to invest in WIFS programmes; and
- ensure a shift in the attitudes and behaviour of WRA that results in regular purchasing and consumption of WIFS.

In Egypt, the communication strategy targeted students and the community message stressed the role of WIFS in terms of mental development, school performance, energy and physical growth. This was reported as being acceptable and convincing. In WIFS programmes where adolescent girls in schools are the target, the following three-tiered communication actions are reported to be effective: school-level activities, reinforcement of messages at the home level, and mobilization of community support.

To promote routine consumption of WIFS and sustain a high level of compliance, it is critical that recipients, and the community, are informed of the benefits of WIFS. The benefits often reported to influence behaviour are those that are readily experienced by WRA following consumption of WIFS. These include improved concentration in school, feeling stronger and less tired, increased energy levels and output in day-to-day work, increased appetite, improved overall capacity to work and earn, better sleep, improved skin appearance, regularization of menstruation, and building of pre-pregnancy health. Communication strategies must encourage sharing of these benefits, through community and peer-group interactions, in order to create a supportive environment for the WIFS programme and to increase demand and compliance. Such a strategy was demonstrated to be effective in the Bihar and Madhya Pradesh WIFS programmes in India.

Recipients should also be informed of side-effects, such as black stools, nausea and vomiting, but care should be taken to present the information on side-effects in such a manner that there is less significance attached to these than the benefits. The tendency to overemphasize side-effects should be discouraged for the following two well-documented reasons: the reported adverse effects are often transitory and the frequency of WIFS side-effects is much lower than with daily doses. Moreover, side-effects decrease over time as reported, for example, in the programmes in Egypt and the Lao People's Democratic Republic.

Advice to WRA to consume WIFS on a full stomach, prior to retiring at night, reduces the incidence of side-effects and should be a part of the communication strategy, as was the case in three Indian programmes (Uttar Pradesh, Gujarat, Madhya Pradesh) and the Lao People's Democratic Republic. For improved iron absorption, the advice to be provided is that supplements should be taken at least two hours after a meal. Such measures have been shown to increase compliance. A compliance survey conducted early in the implementation phase is beneficial in modifying plans and introducing measures to sustain high compliance. Viet Nam's programmes demonstrated that WRA, if convinced at the start of the project through an effective communication strategy, maintain high compliance. It has been well documented by various programmes that high compliance can be achieved, irrespective of supervision, provided recipients are convinced of the benefits of WIFS through an effective communication strategy and a system is in place for monitoring consumption.

Including female front-line workers in programmes as beneficiaries of WIFS has been demonstrated to be a useful social mobilization strategy. Additionally, community-based actions, such as organizing periodic sessions and conducting campaigns to motivate people to buy or use WIFS, are critical in generating a supportive environment. In special situations, such as harvesting season, modifications to the communication strategy need to be introduced, as was done in the programme in Hai Duong Province in Viet Nam, to sustain demand for WIFS and remind busy women to consume IFA supplements every week.

An active effort needs to be made to be vigilant and take timely actions to discourage the spread of any incorrect rumours that may be detrimental to the operation of the WIFS programme. In the programme in Hai Duong Province in Viet Nam, activities were implemented regularly to counteract any negative influences. In Cambodia, rumours that the IFA tablets contained amphetamine to make women work harder and also had a contraceptive effect were handled by addressing these issues through a well-planned communication strategy.

Communication strategies are distinctly different for WIFS programmes where supplements are not supplied free of charge. If WRA are to be mobilized to purchase WIFS, an effective social marketing and social mobilization programme is required. Such a programme needs to be positioned around the four Ps of marketing:

- Product (importance and benefits);
- Price (information on cost and encouragement to buy IFA tablets);
- Place (availability of IFA tablets at all times); and
- Promotion (of the product, price and place, including advertising, packaging, point-of-sale displays and special events).

Experiences of social marketing strategies in Cambodia, the Lao People's Democratic Republic and the Philippines, and in Hai Duong Province in Viet Nam, indicate that the positive positioning of IFA supplements is very effective.

Demand creation through an attractively presented product that appeals to WRA is of prime importance. Additionally, a distinct name and image, promoted through a well-planned communication strategy, increases the acceptance of WIFS. A logo for the product designed around the concept of iron supplements and their impact on health and beauty is well accepted when complemented by a standardized "catchy" message. Logos used in various programmes have included a picture of an attractive "blossoming young woman" or of a beautiful girl holding a rose. To promote the product and reinforce the message, logos and standardized messages may also be printed on varied materials, such as fliers, billboards, banners, etc. In Cambodia's programme, sharing of information on haemoglobin levels was noted to be a factor in motivating secondary-school girls to purchase IFA supplements.

To create demand, communication and social marketing strategies need to be complemented by well-planned social mobilization activities. Experiences reveal that involvement of the community is critical to creating an appropriately supportive environment and for the success and sustainability of WIFS programmes, while mobilization of local leaders is important for successful implementation. The WIFS programme in the Lao People's Democratic Republic indicated that organizing field visits to project sites is useful in generating the interest and support of political leaders. Social mobilization activities there proved effective in securing leadership support from community members, as well as influential members of the community, administrators and politicians. A high-profile programme launch, with involvement of senior administrators and politicians, adds further value to social mobilization efforts. In addition, social mobilization campaigns focusing on women adopting WIFS as a regular habit act as reminders and motivate community members or busy women to purchase and consume tablets. Such promotional reinforcement activities are also important in counteracting any negative influences and trends, such as incorrect information or rumours relating to the routine consumption of supplements.

A fixed-day approach for distribution and consumption of WIFS can be promoted through the communication strategy. This concept was used with great success across all 10 WIFS programmes reviewed. A fixed-day approach has been observed, not only to serve as a good reminder to WRA and the community to consume WIFS, but also to be a very effective programme-management tool. To select a designated WIFS Day, the local situation needs to be taken into consideration. Use of a fixed day for consumption of WIFS addresses the issue of forgetfulness, which has been identified as the major factor adversely influencing compliance. Placing an IFA tablet on a pillow on the fixed day acts as an effective reminder and should be promoted.

> **A fixed-day approach, not only serves as a good reminder to WRA and the community to consume WIFS, but is also a very effective programme-management tool.**

8. Capacity development

> For capacity development, training plans and content need to be formulated based on the identified roles and responsibilities of the various stakeholders in the WIFS programme. Technical information on WIFS should be accurate and standardized. Training should stress, not only technical details, but also skills in the management of supply logistics, use of IEC materials and monitoring. For adolescents, training in family-life education, rather than merely in prevention measures for ID and anaemia, is important in sustaining the interest of trainees. The training plan needs to ensure the building of capacity of at least one selected institution to undertake laboratory testing to monitor the WIFS programme and respond to further requirements, if any.

Ensuring uniform understanding is critical to effective coordination of the health and non-health sectors. It is, therefore, crucial to define the roles and responsibilities of stakeholders, and to identify the knowledge as well as the skills required for effective execution of those responsibilities. Table 6 presents an example of stakeholders and their responsibilities. Development of a training package or training manual is important to facilitate the standardization of information imparted at various levels, including the pharmaceutical and advertising sectors, and to ensure that training provides accurate and relevant information to perform the assigned tasks.

Training content should focus on the importance of preventing ID and anaemia; the benefits of preventing ID; measures for the prevention of ID, including dietary sources of iron; and the significance of WIFS. Additionally, training should put special effort into imparting skills in conducting group and interpersonal counselling, including the use of communication aids. Equally important is training on IFA supply logistics, management of IFA sales and consumption, completion of monitoring forms and analysis of information at the local level, and monitoring of sales and usage of supplements, as well skills in management of funds.

	Table 6: Development of training plans – defining stakeholders and their responsibilities	
I	At government level	Stakeholders - Ministry of Health and Family Welfare; Departments of Health, Nutrition, Secondary Education, Women's Development, Rural and Urban Development; managers of private-sector organizations Responsibilities – Formulate and implement WIFS strategies and policy. Establish a monitoring mechanism. Allocate resources — financial, human and organizational.
II	Nodal professional bodies (public health- or nutrition-related) and research institutes	Responsibilities • Advocacy for according high priority to anaemia prevention and control in WRA. • Technical support in formulation of policy and strategy, education and training of trainers, training of nodal service providers. • Participation in formative research, monitoring and evaluation. • Provision of support for timely action to resolve constraints.
III	Health programme manager	Responsibilities • Training and supervision of staff for effective implementation of plan, using a fixed-day approach for distribution to recipients. • Ensuring timely and regular procurement of supplies and logistics management. • Creation of demand for WIFS and ensuring high compliance. • Monitoring of implementation, including social mobilization and education activities • Periodic checking of compliance through group discussions, etc. • Management of resources.
IV	Education programme manager	Responsibilities • Ensuring the fixed-day strategy is put into operation in schools for adolescent girls. • Establishment of systems for assessment of WIFS supply. Logistics management. • Monitoring of reports on usage and compliance, shared regularly with health department. • Communication strategy on prevention of anaemia through diet and supplements. High compliance of WIFS. • Maintaining ability to undertake family-life education sessions.
V	Health care providers / teachers / community leaders.	Responsibilities • Distribution of IFA supplements. • Effective counselling of WRA to influence behaviour as regards dietary modifications and regular WIFS consumption. • Ensuring teachers and health workers are equipped to undertake family-life education sessions. • Identification of constraints and taking of timely actions to resolve compliance problems. • Monitoring of WIFS supply and consumption.
VI	Adolescent girls in school / out of school and other WRA	Responsibilities • Awareness of the significance of anaemia and its prevention. • Obtaining IFA supplements regularly — institutionalizing a fixed-day system to facilitate regular consumption. • Consuming supplements regularly and managing side-effects. • Reporting constraints to health care providers / teachers — side-effects or inaccessibility of supply.

In the case of adolescent girls, training in how to improve iron status and prevent anaemia could be positioned as a part of family-life education. Such a comprehensive training approach is much more acceptable to adolescent girls, who are at a stage of life where they are curious about a number of issues related to physical changes in their bodies and are also interested in building their self-image and understanding their social environment. Skills in counselling their peer groups should also be a part of the training. The training content could be modified for trainers, including teachers. To encourage question/answer sessions, the use of a "question box" has proved effective, since such a system gives an opportunity to young girls, who are often very shy, to raise questions without revealing their identities.

The training plans must include ensuring the capacity of selected institutions to conduct laboratory tests, such as haemoglobin and serum ferritin estimations.

9. Monitoring

Monitoring of WIFS programmes is critical to effective implementation and high compliance. Simple, standardized individual and group registers for recording supply and compliance have proved effective for monitoring supply, usage and compliance. Individual monitoring cards maintained by consumers are also effective tools for reinforcing messages and act as reminders for consumption of WIFS. In the case of programmes based on social marketing of WIFS, recording sales figures is a useful tool for monitoring supply and usage.

Monitoring details should ideally be included in the planning stage of the WIFS programme. A standardized, user-friendly monitoring format designed to help enter data on supply, distribution and consumption of IFA supplements in minimum time is critical. All four Indian programmes have demonstrated the positive impact monitoring can have on WIFS programmes by improving coverage, reducing drop-outs and increasing WIFS compliance. Monitoring forms in the Gujarat and Bihar programmes are simple, with one red circle against the fixed WIFS day of each week or simply a cluster of four red circles per month. The format focuses on individual monitoring by WRA and entering of information on a monthly basis in a central register.

A number of studies have demonstrated that, in school-based WIFS programmes, individual cards held by WRA are useful. During scaling-up, such a monitoring system is difficult to sustain. However, individual monitoring or compliance cards have proved to be a very effective tool for reinforcing messages on the benefits of regular usage of WIFS and for acting as a reminder to consume WIFS on WIFS Day. Use of such a format therefore plays a significant role in improving compliance, since in three WIFS programmes (Uttar Pradesh and Gujarat in India and the Lao People's Democratic Republic) forgetfulness was reported to be the primary reason for reductions in compliance.

Use of monitoring registers at a class or school level, with information entered each week by each adolescent girl, has also been reported to be practical, simple and acceptable to teachers. In such registers, specific columns are used for recording information on side-effects and reasons for discontinuation of WIFS. The information is very useful in following up cases of low compliance and organizing counselling sessions. Similar monitoring registers are recommended for other institutional set-ups, such as factories or other workplaces. In situations where the implementation strategy has been dovetailed with ongoing programmes for WRA, monitoring information related to WIFS could be linked with existing monitoring systems. The WIFS programme in Egypt indicated that development and use of software for rapid compilation of WIFS monitoring data at the district level can be useful and facilitates problem-solving. In countries where WIFS are promoted for purchase by WRA, pharmaceutical retailers can play an important role in monitoring supply and consumption.

Mechanisms need to be established for review of emerging data in periodic monitoring-committee meetings, with the participation of various stakeholders. In a school situation, formation of a school WIFS committee, with teacher and student representation, has been found to facilitate regular monitoring and appropriate management of the programme. Such a forum helps facilitate regular review and timely action for revisiting intervention strategies and the operational plan. Monitoring mechanisms need to be further strengthened by the inclusion of outcome and impact indicators for the WIFS programme in surveys organized routinely at either the national or regional level.

10. Evaluation

Evaluation should review the effectiveness and constraints of a wide range of WIFS programme components including policy, training, IEC, supply of supplements, system of compliance, assessment, monitoring and cost. Both process and impact indicators should be a part of the evaluation design. Key indicators should be selected based on the local programme situation. The WHO Global Consultation on Weekly Iron and Folic Acid Supplementation for Preventing Anaemia in Women of Reproductive Age recommended annual evaluation for the first five years, with close monitoring considered desirable in the first year.

Evaluation, including process and impact evaluation, should be integrated into the WIFS programme plan from the start. Process evaluation provides information to review the effectiveness and constraints of a strategy, while impact evaluation helps determine if the programme is having the desired impact on haemoglobin levels, anaemia prevalence, iron and folate status and other biological parameters. The laboratory methods used should be standardized. Since the WIFS programme, to a great extent, is dependent upon achievement of behavioural aims and objectives, it is crucial that the evaluation design includes assessment of the knowledge, attitudes and practices of programme agents and beneficiaries, compliance in taking the supplements and cost per recipient. Annual evaluation for the first five years was recommended by the WHO Global Consultation on Weekly Iron and Folic Acid Supplementation for Preventing Anaemia in Women of Reproductive Age (Manila, Philippines, 25-27 April 2007), while close monitoring was considered desirable in the first year. Evaluation conducted early in the implementation phase is beneficial for modification of plans and for making timely strategic shifts in programme implementation. Recommended biological indicators are presented in Annex 4. It should be noted that, as per the recommendations of the Global Consultation, the indicators presented are desirable indicators under ideal conditions. WIFS programme managers, based on programme requirements, can decide which indicators are feasible and desirable.

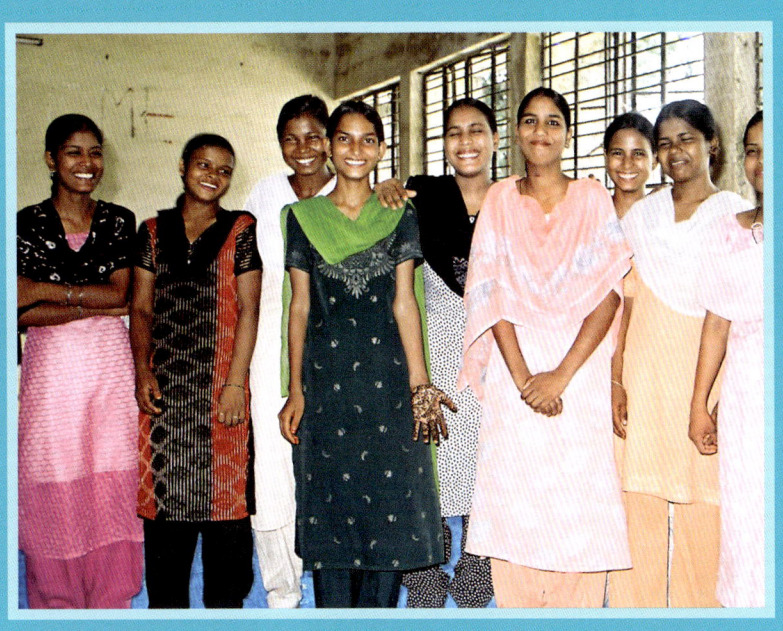

Section III : WIFS programmes — Country case studies

1. India (Bihar)

1.1 Implementation of the Anaemia Control Programme by the education sector

PROJECT AT A GLANCE	
Date of programme	• Phase 1 - March 2000-2002 • Phase 2 - August 2005 – April 2008 • Phase 3 - May 2008 onwards
Location	• Bihar (India)
Number of participants	• Estimated 1 100 088 adolescent girls
Project managed by	• Education Department, with the support of the health sector
Reduction in anaemia rate	• 9.3% in a one-year period
Compliance rate	• 85.2% - 92.2%
Programme costs	• Cost of WIFS programme US$0.32 per adolescent girl/year • Cost of WIFS = US$0.12 per adolescent girl/year

A. Project design

Background

The Anaemia Control Programme in Bihar state, an initiative of the State Government undertaken in collaboration with the United Nations Children's Fund (UNICEF), was launched initially as a pilot project on 24 March 2000 in two districts of the state — Gaya and Muzaffarpur. Over eight years, the project was expanded to cover the entire Bihar state of 38 districts.

WRA target group and programme roles and responsibilities

In the pilot phase, initial effort was made to reach only girls in schools; later a strategy was adopted to reach girls out of school. During the pilot phase of 2000-2002, a total of 79 590 schoolgirls (standards VI to XII) and 191 070 non-school girls from the two districts were reached. The overall compliance rate over the two years of implementation was reported to be 70% in one district and 72% in the other.

In each district, a district support team of two persons and three field coordinators worked with the Education Department and a network of identified schoolteachers. The district support teams were responsible for conducting block-level meetings and orientation of principals, schoolteachers and village leaders, as well as monitoring inputs at the school level. Field Coordinators were responsible for providing programmatic support to ensure smooth operation of the project activities, including planning, demand creation, supply, community awareness and progressive recording of coverage. Teachers were motivators, guides and promoters for the targeted adolescent girls in schools as well as girls not in school.

A special effort was made to reach out-of-school girls, using a peer-to-peer or girl-to-girl approach. "Motivator girls" were selected in each school and were given the responsibility of reaching out-of-school girls with weekly IFA supplements and ensuring compliance. These activities were coordinated by the Integrated Child Development Services (ICDS) or Anganwadi Centres.

Monitoring system

The monitoring system involved recording the consumption of IFA supplements at two levels: at an individual level by the girls themselves, who filled in the individual compliance cards retained by teachers; and by teachers, in school registers especially designed for the WIFS programme. Information on the IFA supplies received and consumed, as well as the supply requirements for subsequent months, was entered in the register at the school level.

B. Process and progress

Programme launch

> Partnerships between a wide range of strategic players were considered essential to the success of the Anaemia Control Programme, with a primary focus on WIFS.

The inaugural function was attended by senior district and block officials from the Health, Education and Child Development Departments, as well as the media. Partnerships between strategic players were considered essential to the success of the Anaemia Control Programme, with a primary focus on WIFS. The high-profile launch was therefore used as an opportunity to highlight the significance of the partnerships between the three primary sectors and to ensure that the public health problem of anaemia, including the significance of the WIFS programme, was accorded high priority. Media reports on the WIFS project further facilitated generation of awareness about the project.

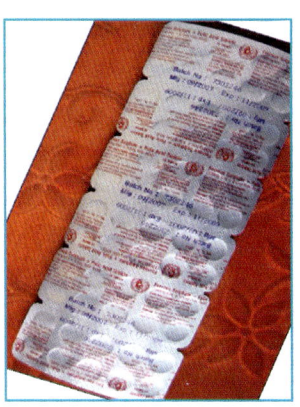

Blister packs of iron and folic acid tablets

IFA supply

The IFA supply was procured by UNICEF. The non-sugar-coated IFA tablets were coated with a brown-red film and contained 100 mg of elemental iron in the form of ferrous sulphate and 0.5 mg of folic acid per tablet. The composition of the tablet was identical to that used by pregnant mothers in the national programme. There were 10 tablets in each blister pack and 100 such packs were provided in a box. The cost of 100 tablets was INR11.40 or US$0.24. A year's supply of 52 non-sugar-coated tablets for an adolescent girl therefore cost just US$0.12. Each girl consumed an IFA tablet once a week in the presence of nodal teachers on the day fixed for distribution of the tablets. Girls were instructed not to consume the IFA supplements on an empty stomach and were informed of possible transitory side effects, such as nausea, change in stool colour and constipation, etc.

IEC activities

The educational activities focused on generating awareness regarding the high prevalence of anaemia as a public health problem and simple, well-proven preventive measures, including dietary sources of iron and WIFS. Educational and promotional activities included wall-writing campaigns, prabhat pheri or community awareness-raising walks by schoolchildren, drawing slogans and essay writing competitions. Information was also broadcast through television and radio networks and newspaper advertisements. Village education committees were also informed and equipped with information materials to help mobilize parents and the community.

The educational and promotional activities for WIFS, in their initial phase, concentrated on environment building and social mobilization on the issue of

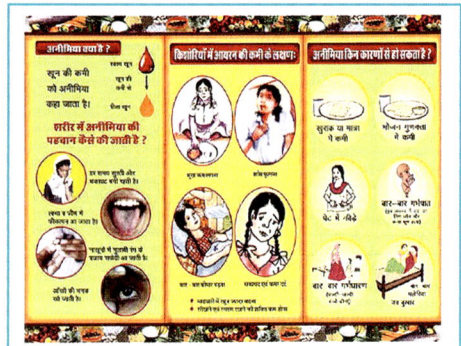 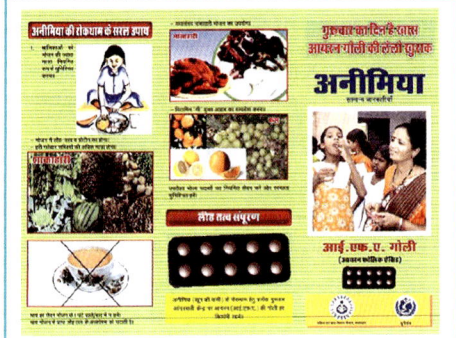

IEC materials used

anaemia. Awareness campaigns were organized. The community was informed about the causes, effects and prevention of anaemia, with an emphasis on:

- adoption of correct dietary practices;
- creating demand for IFA supplements; and
- promoting weekly consumption of WIFS.

Parents of adolescent girls were informed of the significance of WIFS in various forums, including village meetings, women's group meetings and community discussions. Effort was also made to address any misconceptions or rumours regarding WIFS.

Training

Six training modules were developed and used, with each module designed to target a specific group, such as: district-level heads, block-level functionaries, master trainers, nodal teachers, school-attending adolescent girls and village/community-level communicators. The training focused on anaemia prevention and control, the roles and responsibilities of teachers and girls in implementing the project, and appropriate techniques to be followed for the storage and distribution of IFA tablets and for recording the supply of IFA and compliance.

Scaling up – Phase two

Based on the pilot project's success over two years in two districts, the project was extended to about 50% of the districts in the state in its second phase (August 2005 — April 2008) with a focus on school-attending girls, aged 10-19 years, in standards VIII to XII. Sixteen of the total 38 districts were covered. The objective of the WIFS programme was "to support longer years of progressive schooling and improve their quality of life by improving nutrition-health and education status". The intervention package in the second phase comprised WIFS, family-life education and an additional component of administering deworming medication (albendazole 400mg) twice a year. IFA tablets, as in phase one, were supplied by UNICEF.

IFA was administered, in all 16 districts, every Wednesday during the first period. The girls were instructed to consume the IFA tablets on a full stomach and to use water for swallowing. The adolescent girls were instructed not to drink tea or coffee prior to or after consumption. Education on anaemia was, in fact, made part of the broader curriculum of family-life education. Unlike in the demonstration phase, the Secondary Education Unit of the Department of Education and not the Social Welfare Department was in overall charge of the implementation and

> The objective of the WIFS programme was "to support longer years of progressive schooling and improve their quality of life by improving nutrition-health and education status".

monitoring procedures throughout the second phase. Since this intervention was not part of the routine education system, the roles and responsibilities of the education sector at state, district, block and village level were clearly defined, as outlined below:

Level	Partner	Role
State	Director of Education or Human Resource Development (HRD)	Overall supervision of the programme
District	District Education Officer	Programme review and supervision of programme with respect to training, IFA supplementation, monitoring, compilation of data at district level, orientation of school staff
School	Headmaster and nodal teachers	Implementation of programme: - provision of supplements to girls, - Orientation and counselling of girls on consequences of anaemia, with special focus on nutritional and health status and educational performance, Counselling on dietary modification, - Compilation of school-level data and preparation of reports, - Assessment of requirements of IFA supplies and - Organization of promotional activities, etc.

Additionally, information on family-life education, including important social issues, such as prevention of adolescent marriage and conception, and the significance of educating girls, also formed an important component of the training in the second phase. Training also emphasized the development of skills for implementation of various components of the programme viz. logistical management of IFA supplements, counselling for the development of positive attitudes regarding adolescent health and WIFS consumption, monitoring and recording compliance, and estimation of haemoglobin levels. A technical team was selected and trained by a non-government organization and was linked with a pathology department for support in the estimation of haemoglobin levels using a cyanmethaemoglobin method.

Consumption was supervised by peer leaders or nodal teachers. The demand-creation strategy, described above for the demonstration phase, continued to be implemented. Regular counselling sessions were organized by teachers for both girls and their parents. For girls not in school, counselling sessions were organized by the village governing committee (Panchayati Raj Institution or PRI) members, as well as community volunteers associated with other ongoing development programmes in the region. These community volunteers were generally young men and women who acted as facilitators for school-level activities. In each district, eight volunteers were trained to provide support in schools for the organization of promotional activities, ensuring completion of teacher training and formation or revival of parents-teachers associations, and estimation of IFA supplement requirements. The focus was on convincing girls, as well as community and family members associated with adolescent girls, of the benefits of WIFS. Educational information highlighted the importance of improving the nutrition of adolescents and preventing iron deficiency and anaemia, the benefits of WIFS and the significance of delaying the age of marriage and conception. Educational and promotional activities were conducted in community gatherings organized in villages. During these community gatherings, girls were given the opportunity to share positive experiences related to regular use of WIFS. A set of information and educational materials were developed, consisting of a set of four posters, information folders and booklets, as well as a collection of stories, games and songs. A short, catchy message on anaemia prevention and control was standardized and printed on educational materials as well as on compliance cards, registers and booklets for adolescent girls both in and out of school.

As the monitoring system and forms experimented with in the demonstration phase had proved to be effective, they were used in the expansion phase. The forms used at both school and district levels also included information on the IFA supply received and estimated future requirements. These forms were submitted on a monthly basis by each school to the district authorities and finally to the State Department of Education. Information received on supply requirements formed the basis for procurement and distribution of IFA supplement supplies to schools by district authorities.

Programme partners at all levels (District Education Officers, headmasters and nodal teachers) in each district helped in monitoring programme interventions and made an active effort to address side-effects. The progress of the WIFS programme was monitored at six-monthly intervals by the District Coordination Committee, comprising district and block officers of education, health and ICDS. To ensure the WIFS project was given high priority, a district-level meeting was held every month under the chairmanship of the district magistrate.

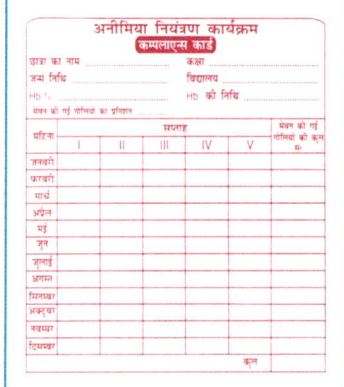

Individual compliance monitoring card

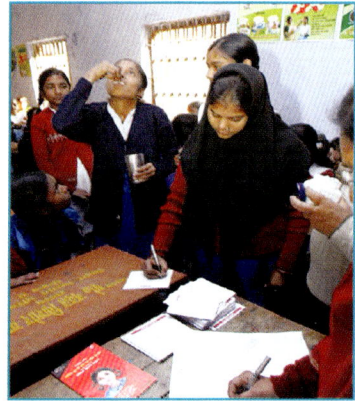

Use of class register for monitoring and capacity-building session at school

The impact of WIFS on adolescent girls, in school, over a period of 52 weeks, was studied. Findings indicated that 85.2%-92.2% had complied with WIFS. Interesting benefits of WIFS were reported (Table 7) and these were used for counselling sessions.

Table 7: Changes experienced after IFA supplementation, as reported by girls (N=1700)	
Changes experienced after IFA supplementation	Percentage (%)
Feeling less tired	28.7
No problem of breathlessness	23.6
Feeling more active	45.4
Fall sick less often	41.1
Better concentration in studies	48.4
Participation in sports	24.5
More involvement in domestic chores	31.6
Others	5.6
No change	7.5

In the second year of implementation, over a period of 52 weeks, anaemia prevalence decreased from the 93.1% reported at baseline (4653 girls) in 2005 to 84.4% in 2006-2007 (1500 girls). This difference is significant ($p<0.001$).

In the second phase, 0.3 million adolescent girls from 1348 high schools were covered. The cost per beneficiary was estimated to be INR 15 (US$0.32) / girl / year, with WIFS costing INR 6 (US$0.12) / girl / year. Due to the progress and impact of the WIFS programme, the third phase of the Adolescent Anaemia Control Programme was launched to cover the entire Bihar state of 38 districts, from mid-2008. The following lessons, learnt from the first 52 weeks of implementation, were taken into consideration in completion of the second phase and planning for the third phase of whole-state coverage:

- Use a fixed- day approach (Wednesday of every week).
- Clearly define roles and responsibilities for the education sector.
- Streamline supply, with involvement of the health sector.
- Ensure a regular and good quality supply.
- Increase acceptance of the WIFS programme and compliance by interacting with the community and emphasising association with reduction in lethargy and improvement in concentration at school.
- Inform parents, teachers and beneficiaries of benefits, as well as preparing them to manage and treat side-effects.
- Involve female teachers to increase acceptance of the programme.

Scaling-up – Phase three

In the third phase, the project intervention package continues to consist of WIFS, biannual deworming and family-life education. The Education Department has overall responsibility for the Anaemia Control Programme and is implementing the WIFS programme in coordination with the health sector. Accordingly, an operational plan of action is being developed to reach girls aged 12-20 years, with the State Government taking over the responsibility for supplying IFA supplements to the entire state from its own resources under the National Rural Health Mission (NRHM). The cost per beneficiary is estimated to have been reduced to INR 11.80 (US$0.28) per year. This includes the cost of biannual deworming, WIFS (52 IFA non-sugar-coated tablets costing US$0.12 per beneficiary), IEC materials, monitoring forms and monitoring registers. The cost of WIFS is about 50% of the total programme cost per girl annually.

1.2 Lessons learnt

- WIFS intervention, combined with biannual deworming and family-life education, is critical to reducing anaemia in adolescent girls. The annual estimated cost per beneficiary with such an intervention package is estimated to be only about US$0.32 per year.
- The Anaemia Control Programme for adolescent girls in school requires the Department of Education to take primary responsibility. To gain support from the Education Department, implications of anaemia on school performance must be clearly stated. It is essential to define the roles and responsibilities of the Education Department in implementing the WIFS programme. Collaboration with other departments will contribute to creating the right demand and environment for the WIFS programme.

- Reaching out-of-school adolescent girls and encouraging acceptance of WIFS requires a planned, intensive effort to interact with both the girls and also the community. Introduction of a girl-to-girl approach to mobilize girls for WIFS consumption and organization of centre-based distribution for IFA supplements increases the reach and scope of supervised consumption.
- The fixed-day strategy used for IFA distribution facilitates overall WIFS programme implementation, including mobilization, distribution, supervision and monitoring by teachers or other front-line workers or village leaders or volunteers.
- Teachers are effective motivators of girls. Assigning the task of the WIFS programme to female teachers increases acceptance.
- Overall compliance of WIFS has been over 80%. A communication strategy, using the sharing of positive experiences regarding the benefits of IFA supplements in a community gathering is critical to the development of supportive environments.
- Instructions not to consume IFA supplements on an empty stomach possibly contributed significantly to reduced side-effects and increasing compliance.
- The fixed-day strategy used for IFA distribution facilitates overall WIFS programme implementation, including mobilization, distribution, supervision and monitoring by teachers or other front-line workers or village leaders or volunteers.
- Teachers are effective motivators of girls. Assigning the task of the WIFS programme to female teachers increases acceptance.
- Overall compliance of WIFS has been over 80%. A communication strategy, using the sharing of positive experiences regarding the benefits of IFA supplements in a community gathering is critical to the development of supportive environments.
- Instructions not to consume IFA supplements on an empty stomach possibly contributed significantly to reduced side-effects and increasing compliance.
- Monitoring actions are important at two levels — individual compliance cards to be completed by each adolescent girl and retained by teachers, and school registers to be completed by nodal teachers. School registers should also include information on the number of IFA tablets provided and consumed by students and monthly supply requirements.
- Formation of district training teams of five to eight persons is desirable. These volunteers can support the Education Department and the teachers' network in undertaking defined tasks, such as block-level meetings, orientation of teachers and village leaders, and monitoring support. The sustainability of this approach needs to be critically studied.
- Active effort is needed to manage the side-effects of WIFS. This can be done to a great extent by educating and involving parents, teachers and beneficiaries.
- Creation of demand for WIFS for non-school-attending girls requires a strategy beyond the school channel. It is therefore crucial to dovetail the WIFS programme with multiple channels of distribution, including other centre-based development activities, e.g. the adolescent scheme of the Directorate of Integrated Child Development Services (ICDS).

References

1) *Control of nutritional anaemia in school going adolescent girl: experiences in Bihar.* Government of Bihar and UNICEF.
2) Saiyed F., Nutrition Specialist, UNICEF Patna field office report (2008).

1.3 Bihar (India) WIFS Programme — A summary

Time framework & coverage	Age group	Anaemia prevalence	Intervention package	Nodal implementing agencies	Impact	Current status
• Phase 1 - 2000-2002. Covered two districts or 79 590 SG and 191 670 OSG*. • Phase 2 - August 2005 – April 2008. Covered 16 of the 38 districts (300 088) • Phase 3 - May 2008 onwards. Entire state (38 districts) covered. About 800 000 adolescent girls	VI-XII class, 10-19 years VII-XII class, 12-19/20 years	95.1% adolescent girls anaemic	• WIFS • Deworming (400 mg albendazole) • Family-life education, including anaemia prevention and promotion of iron-rich food	• Education sector, with support of health sector • Directorate of Integrated Child Development Services (ICDS)	• Anaemia prevalence decreased from 93.1% to 84.4% in a period of one year – a significant decrease of 9.3%.	• Control of anaemia in adolescent girls included in the 11th five-year development plan of India • State Nutrition Policy to include WIFS programme • National Rural Health Mission (NRHM) - all high schools in 38 districts (estimated adolescent girls 800 000) are being covered since mid-2008.

Supply and consumption of WIFS

Composition, packaging and supply procurement	Cost	Specific approach used	Specific consumption instructions	IFA Supply to recipients		Supervision during WIFS consumption
				Free / purchased	Access	
IFA = 100 mg of elemental iron as ferrous sulphate and 0.5 mg of folic acid, non-sugar-coated, brown-red, blister packs of 10-30. Composition same as for pregnant women. UNICEF supply (in phases 1 and 2) and government supply (phase 3)	• Cost of WIFS programme = US $ 0.32 per adolescent girl / year. • Cost of WIFS = US $ 0.12 / year (38% of the total WIFS project cost)	Fixed day – Wednesday of every week (first period in school).	• Do not consume IFA on an empty stomach, but after meal. • Use water for swallowing. • No tea or coffee prior to or after consumption of IFA supplements.	• Free of cost (SG* + OSG*). • UNICEF supply in first and second phases. • Government supply planned in phase 3.	Teachers distribute to schoolgirls on fixed WIFS days.	Nodal teachers supervise adolescent girls in schools.

* SG = School-going (girls) OSG = Out-of-school girls

Efforts to increase compliance (IEC / Social mobilization / Strategy)

Positive attributes / benefits experienced	Side-effects reported and managed	Supplement-promotion strategy	Compliance
• Efforts made to address any misconceptions or rumours. • Benefits reported: feeling less tired, no breathlessness, feeling more active, fall sick less often, better concentration in studies, participation in sports, increased involvement in domestic chores.	• Active efforts to address side-effects – nausea, change in stool colour, constipation. • Parents, teachers and girls trained to manage side-effects • Advised to take supplements on full stomach.	• Emphasis on the regular intake of iron / folic acid supplements, on reduction of lethargy and increased concentration at school. Reduction in absences from school, drop-outs. • Education on anaemia part of family-life education. • Local community-based activities (community walks with raising of slogans) complemented by mass media activities (TV / radio / advertisements). Focus on adoption of correct dietary practices and promoting weekly consumption. • During community gatherings, sharing of positive benefits encouraged. • Counselling sessions for girls and their parents on WIFS and dietary sources of iron and inhibitors of iron absorption. • Village governing committee (PRI) involved in counselling sessions. • Information and educational materials: - Posters, information folders, booklets, stories, games, songs. • Messages on anaemia prevention standardized and printed on educational materials, as well as on compliance cards, registers and booklets.	• Compliance 85.2%-92.2%. • Regular supply of supplements and fixed-day strategy.

Training and monitoring

Training	Monitoring Individual cards / registers etc	Other positive contributing factors

Focus of training – anaemia, WIFS and dietary management
• Anaemia prevention and control:
  - awareness about anaemia and its consequences;
  - benefits of WIFS programme.
• Understanding roles and responsibilities.
• Implementation:
  - logistical management - techniques of storage, distribution and recording, supply and compliance;
  - counselling and data on positive attributes of IFA;
  - monitoring and recording;
  - addressing side-effects.
• Six training modules – district heads, block-level functionaries, master trainers, nodal teachers, school-going adolescent girls, village communicators.
	• Individual cards for girls.
	• Registers for class records on WIFS. School registers to record IFA supply received/ consumed and monthly supply requirements.
	• District coordination committee – monitoring every six months.
	• UNICEF extender + eight volunteers in each district help to monitor programme.
		• Department of Education was the nodal department. In future, the role of health is envisaged to include streamlining IFA supply.
		• Roles and responsibilities of the education sector (district-, block- and village-levels) defined at the planning stage.

2. India (Gujarat)

2.1 Scaling Up the Adolescent Girls Anaemia Control Programme through weekly iron-folic acid supplementation (WIFS)

PROJECT AT A GLANCE	
Date of programme	• Pilot project – June 2001 – Dec 2004 • Scaled up – 2005 onwards
Location	• Gujarat (India)
Number of participants	• Estimated 1 265 475 adolescent girls in and out of school
Project managed by	• Health and Education Departments
Reduction in anaemia rate	• 28.8% in a one-year period
Compliance rate	• 89% in schoolgirls and 94% in out-of-school girls
Programme costs	• Cost of WIFS programme US$0.32 per adolescent girl/year • Cost of WIFS supplements US$0.15/girl/year

A. Project design

Background

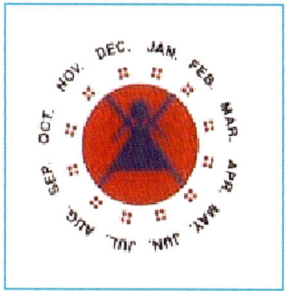

The State Government of Gujarat, a western region of India, in collaboration with Baroda Medical College, and with UNICEF assistance, launched the three-year pilot project "Adolescent Girls Anaemia Reduction Project" on 28 June 2001. The project was launched in the Vadodara district, following a baseline survey, to address the serious situation of anaemia. In 2005, the project was scaled up to cover all 25 districts of the state, reaching an estimated 1 265 475 girls. The logo on the left was used for the project.

Baseline survey

A baseline survey was undertaken in the district of Vadodara, Gujarat, among girls aged 12-19 years. The survey focused on the prevalence of anaemia, the status of iron deficiency, and dietary habits regarding taking iron- and vitamin-rich foods, as well as the knowledge, attitudes and practices regarding anaemia and iron deficiency and the proposed preventive measure of WIFS. It was noted that 74.7% girls were anaemic and, overall, about 50% of girls were found to have low iron stores. The severity of anaemia in girls aged 12-19 years increased with age; iron depletion was highest among girls aged 18-19 years. The baseline survey also showed that 97% of adolescent girls were willing to consume WIFS when offered the supplements in a school setting.

Project goals

A Project Support Unit was established in the Department of Preventive and Social Medicine at the district-based medical college for technical support, research, documentation and overall monitoring of the project. UNICEF provided financial assistance. The goal of the project was to present the State Government with an effective, operational district-level strategy to reduce anaemia prevalence among adolescent girls through two primary interventions: consumption of WIFS under supervision and improved dietary practices. The intervention did not include deworming or family-life education. The aim of the pilot project was primarily to institutionalize a programme for adolescent girls in the state with a focus on provision of WIFS and nutrition education to increase iron intake. The launch of the project was organized as a high-profile event, since the involvement of policy-makers was considered critical right from the start of the project to achieve the stated goal.

Target group

The project was implemented primarily for adolescent girls in school. In the second phase, effort was also made to reach girls out of school. A total of 426 secondary or high schools (standards 8-12) of the district were covered by the District Health Department in collaboration with the Education Department.

During its three-year period, the pilot project was implemented in 410 of the 426 schools and covered 65 000 adolescent schoolgirls. The coverage of out-of-school girls was rather low in the first year, with only 75 schools (18%) taking part in the strategy. A total of 12 067 schoolgirls were covered and they reached only 9536 OSG. In fact, as per the strategy, each of the 65 000 schoolgirls was expected to reach three such OSG or a total of about 195 000 girls.

Programme roles and responsibilities

The health and education sectors had joint responsibility for planning and implementing the Adolescent Girls Anaemia Control Programme through WIFS. The Health Department's responsibilities were defined as:

- ensuring a timely supply of IFA supplements;
- training school teachers;
- monitoring IFA supply; and
- providing technical inputs from district to school level.

The Education Department was responsible for implementing project activities at the school level. In each school, two teachers were selected and put in charge of the anaemia programme. Teachers were responsible for providing supplements to girls, supervising, monitoring and recording consumption of WIFS in registers, imparting nutrition education and encouraging girls to recognize and consume WIFS regularly. Schoolteachers were trained to understand the importance of addressing the problem of anaemia and to undertake the task of monitoring progress. A district-level coordination committee, comprising district education and health officials, contributed towards strengthening joint ownership of the programme by the Health and Education Departments.

Monitoring

Monitoring was undertaken at the following four levels, each using different types of recording formats: individual, class, school and cluster levels. At the individual level, a self-compliance card was introduced. Adolescent girls were trained to mark a cross against each week the supplement was consumed. Self-monitoring at this level played an important role in motivating regular consumption, as well as in sustaining a high level of compliance. The compliance card was used regularly by 50% of girls for self-monitoring. At the class level, monitoring registers were used and information regarding the monthly consumption of each girl and the

> The aim of the pilot project was primarily to institutionalize a programme for adolescent girls in the state with a focus on provision of WIFS and nutrition education to increase iron intake.

class overall was entered by a class monitor or a class teacher. Each class's weekly consumption report was then compiled by each school under the leadership of the principal and sent to the District Education Officer. Reports from a cluster of schools were compiled and reviewed by an education inspector, who visited schools to address any emerging issues. These cluster-level reports were then sent to the Project Support Unit on a monthly basis. It was noted that about 70% of schools sent monitoring reports regularly. No incentives were built into the project, but monitoring by the Project Support Unit, combined with the coordination meeting, appear to have contributed to functioning monitoring mechanisms.

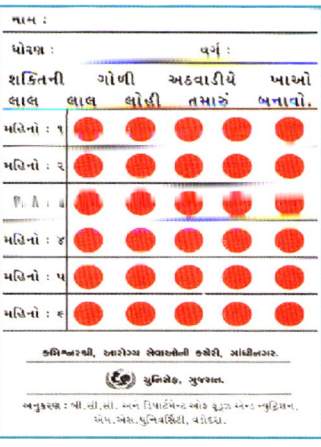
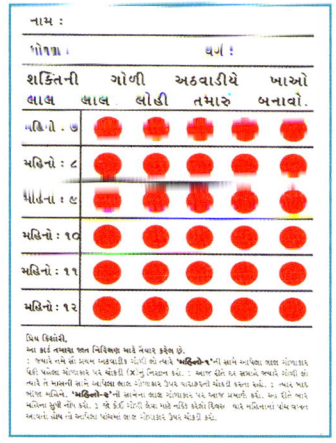

Monitoring card (front)   Monitoring card (back)

A district-level Coordination Committee reviewed project progress at monthly meetings and took necessary actions. The Committee consisted of officials from both the Health and Education Departments (District Education Officers, Chief District Health Officer, Project Coordinator and medical college personnel). Dual representation from the Departments of Health and Education facilitated improved coordination and resulted in strengthening the joint ownership of the project. A monthly magazine for teachers and principals reported the progress of the project, as well as the significance of WIFS. Additionally, information on the project was disseminated periodically through publication of articles in magazines pertaining to health.

B. Process and progress

IFA supply

The composition of non-sugar coated tablets was identical to that used in the national programme for pregnant women. Each tablet contained 100mg of elemental iron and 0.5 mg of folic acid. Support was sought from the Indian Medical Association, a professional body, to give WIFS political and technical recognition. Meetings to gain the support of the district administration and school network and to sensitize them to the public health issue of ID were held with district authorities as well as district-level associations of principals and teachers. Moreover, district health and education persons were involved in the project right from the planning stage.

To ensure a timely supply of IFA supplements, a logistical system was developed, with joint involvement of the education and health sectors. Schools, on the basis of school-monitoring reports, assessed their supply requirements for IFA

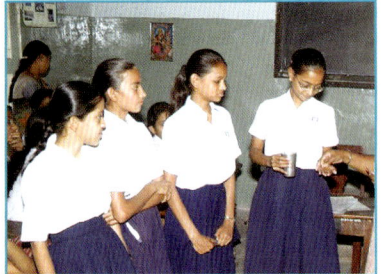 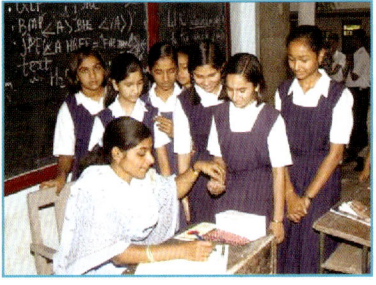 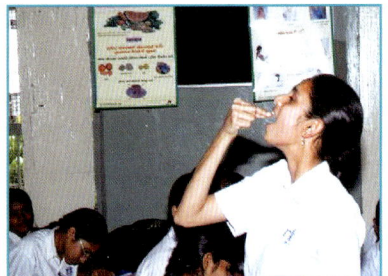

Supervised distribution of IFA supplements to girls.

Schoolgirls queue up for IFA supplements. The teacher records information on consumption.

An adolescent girl consuming an IFA supplement in class.

supplements. Requests for IFA supplies received from schools were put together by the District Education Department, who requested and procured the supply from the District Health Department. The District Education Department arranged for the supply of IFA supplements to be forwarded to individual schools. The Health Department had overall responsibility for the IFA supply and therefore monitored the functioning of the IFA supply chain at least twice a year (Figure 1).

Figure 1: Supply of IFA tablets to schools

Compliance

A fixed-day approach was used for WIFS. Every Wednesday, the IFA supplement was made available to schoolgirls. Wednesday was selected as the most appropriate day since, in consultation with project staff and the community, it was noted that religious fasting was commonly not observed on this day. Therefore, it was expected to be the day of least resistance to consuming the supplements.

Through the school system, a strategy called the "girl-to-girl approach" was initiated to reach out-of-school girls (OSG). Each girl in school was encouraged to reach three OSG and also supervise WIFS consumption. The OSG were instructed to consume tablets every Wednesday, since it was considered the most suitable day for ensuring regular consumption. Only 75 of the 426 schools participated in the girl-to-girl approach. A total of 12 067 girls from these schools reached 9536 girls who were not in school. Additionally, non-government organizations, such as Baroda Citizen's Council, actively participated in WIFS to OSG under supervision. In urban areas, Integrated Child Development Services (ICDS) were also involved in reaching OSG through the Adolescent Girls Scheme, which is referred to as *Kishori Shakti Yojana* or KSY.

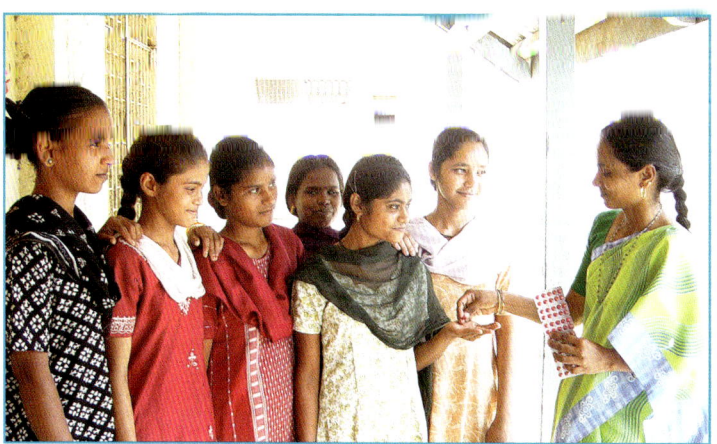

Anganwadi worker giving IFA supplements to adolescent girls

Evaluation findings revealed that the printed materials were read by most of the girls, but their understanding and retention of the message was comparatively low.

IEC activities

To promote consumption of IFA supplements, two types of IEC materials were given to schools: brochures for girls (one per girl) and teachers (one per teacher), and posters (two sets per school). Teachers, as per the guidelines provided during training, displayed posters. Additionally, two copies of an information booklet entitled *20 Frequently asked questions (FAQs) on anaemia* were also provided to each school. The availability and utilization of the IEC materials, as well as the recall of messages, was evaluated using structured forms. Evaluation findings revealed that the printed materials were read by most of the girls, but their understanding and retention of the message was comparatively low. For example, 87.2% of the girls who received the brochure had read it, while 56.3% did not respond when asked to recall three messages from the brochure. It was interesting to note that 99% of those who responded recalled at least one correct message. Therefore school-level activities, including slogan competitions, drawing, debates etc., were introduced in schools. Such activities also generated a lot of interest in the WIFS project in the community.

Training

To ensure effective implementation, medical officers were equipped as trainers and they in turn trained teachers. The interactive training included technical information as well as skill-based training on management of logistics, use of IEC materials, entering data on compliance and side-effects of WIFS on monitoring forms, analysis of monitoring reports, and using emerging information to organize follow-up.

Compliance

Based on the monthly compliance reports, the average compliance, following 17 months of implementation in schools, was reported to be about 89%, while the average compliance reported in OSG over a period of one year was 94%.

Following a year of implementation, 1905 girls were questioned regarding their usage of WIFS during the summer vacation. It was noted that 92.8% of girls had received IFA tablets during the summer vacation, but only 72.1% had consumed them. The most common reason given for not taking WIFS during the summer vacation, reported by 16.3% of girls, was forgetfulness.

Using an open-ended questionnaire, over 2700 girls were interviewed on the side-effects and benefits of WIFS. Initially 29.7% of schoolgirls had reported side-effects, which fell to 14.3% by the end of the year. The most common side-effects reported were abdominal pain, vomiting, giddiness and nausea. These symptoms were often associated with taking the supplement on an empty stomach. The side-effects declined when girls were advised to consume tablets after food. The benefits of taking WIFS were experienced by 50.7% of girls. The most common benefits were: increased work capacity (21.9%), improved or redder blood (16.4%), improved health (7.2%), and decreased pallor (5.1%).

Evaluation

An evaluation was undertaken after one year of implementation to study the change in the haematinic status of the girls and the programme's impact on their knowledge regarding anaemia and its control. The evaluation assessed rural, tribal and urban schools and the same 30 schools selected for the baseline survey. The sample size selected for the evaluation study was 3000. All those girls who were in the baseline study and were still in school were selected on a priority basis. Anaemia prevalence, following one year of implementation, had decreased significantly ($p < 0.05$) from 74.7% to 53.2% in schoolgirls, a reduction of 20.5%, which was statistically significant (Figure 2). In paired data analysis of 1016 adolescent girls, a similar statistically significant decrease from 74.2% to 53.5% was noted.

Figure 2: Change in Anaemia Prevalence

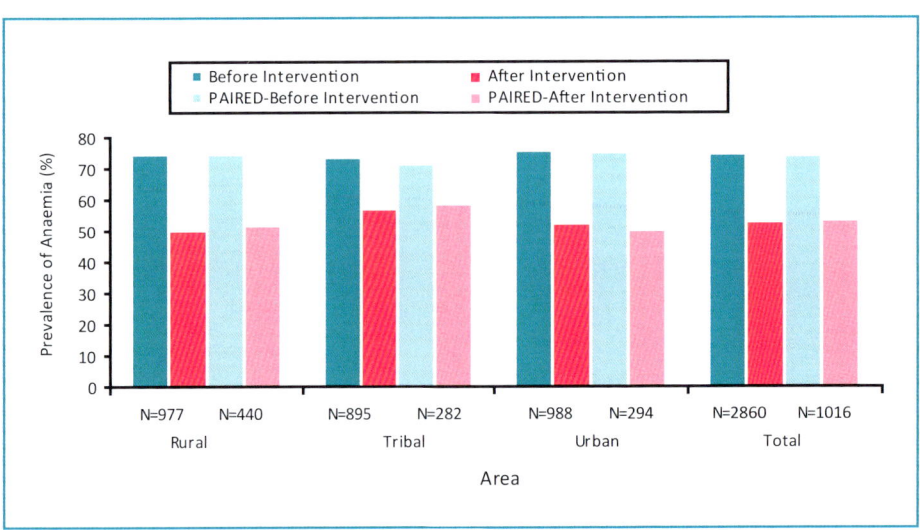

One year of the WIFS programme resulted in converting 13 000 anaemic girls to non-anaemic status.

The changes in the percentage prevalence of anaemia before and after intervention for paired and non-paired analysis was significant (p<0.05) for rural, tribal, urban and total schools.

One year of the WIFS programme therefore resulted in converting 13 000 anaemic girls to non-anaemic status. In tribal areas, with a particularly high percentage of thalassaemia, a 16% reduction was observed. The proportion of girls with normal iron levels increased from 25.3% to 46.8% — an increase of 85% from the baseline level, while severe anaemia prevalence decreased from 1.6% to 0.5% —a decrease of 68% (Figure 3). The proportion of girls with low serum ferritin levels (% below 12ng/ml) declined from 49.7% to 39.4%, indicating a clear improvement. The median ferritin values improved across all ages, with the greatest improvement in rural areas and the least improvement in tribal areas.

Figure 3: Severity of anaemia before and after intervention

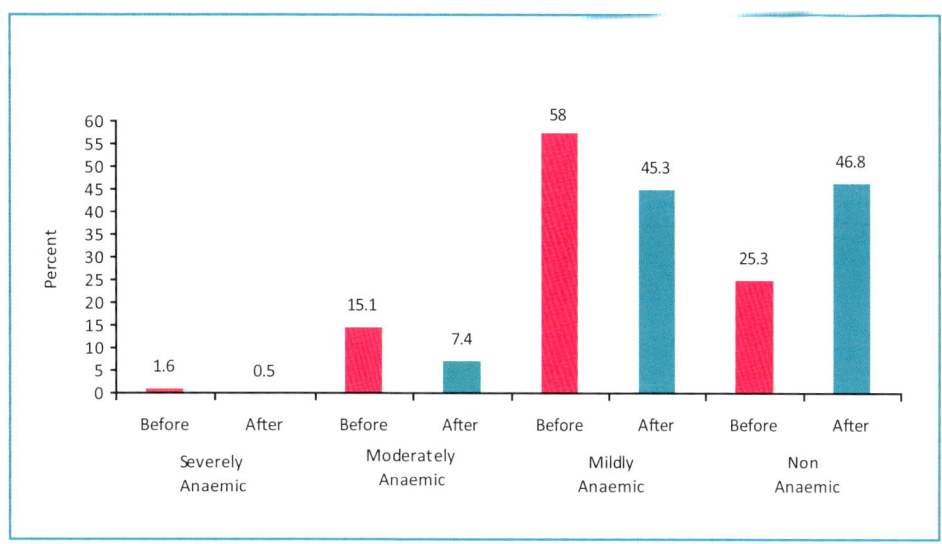

The pilot project revealed that the strategy for reaching adolescent girls in schools through the Education Department, with collaboration from the health sector, was effective. About one quarter of the total number of adolescent girls were effectively reached and addressed the issue of iron deficiency and anaemia. In schools, the support of parents and teachers was found to be of critical importance to schoolgirls.

Reaching girls who were out of school (OSG) was crucial since they formed three quarters of the adolescent population. Under the trial approach of schoolgirls reaching out to non-schoolgirls, success was limited. Only 20% of the schoolgirls who participated in the programme could actually initiate actions for OSG, and less than 50% of targeted OSG were reached. However, the average compliance reported over a period of 11 months was high, at about 94%. Less than 1% of girls stopped taking WIFS because of side-effects or migration. Experimenting with alternative approaches, such as linking the programme with the ongoing Adolescent Girls Scheme of the Integrated Child Development Services (ICDS) or with an NGO was proposed to reach girls out of school.

Scaling up

By December 2004, based on the success of the demonstration project in Vadodara District, it was planned to take the anaemia programme to scale, with the support of UNICEF and the Micronutrient Initiative (MI), in phases in all 25 districts of the state. Between 2005 and 2007, UNICEF and MI support of supply, IEC and monitoring costs was reduced gradually as supply and financial support from the State Government of Gujarat was increased. Since 2008, the Anaemia Control Programme, including provision of IFA supplements, has been totally managed by the State Government of Gujarat. The yearly estimated unit cost per adolescent girl per year is US$0.14 (including the cost of IFA supply, monitoring forms for classes and schools, and brochures for girls in standards 8-12) with an additional cost of IEC materials for schools, every third year, of US$0.01 per girl.

More than one million adolescent girls (almost 99% of those enrolled), in standards 8-12 (14-18 years), from 7663 secondary schools across the state are covered under the National Rural Health Mission (NRHM), with the joint support of the health and education sectors (Figure 4). The Health Department procures and distributes IFA supplements to schools via the Primary Health Centre (PHC) every year. About 71 000 teachers are involved and supervise administration of WIFS on a fixed day—Wednesday. The Education Department monitors compliance and is also responsible for recording information and compiling data on supply and compliance from school to state level. The Education Department shares compliance reports with the Health Department at district and state levels.

Reaching OSG remains a challenge. OSG are being covered primarily through the Adolescent Girls Scheme or KSY of ICDS. Efforts are being made to increase coverage of OSG in partnership with NGOs, such as Sumul Dairy and the Tribhuvan Das Foundation. By mid-2009, 265 475 OSG, only 19 % of the total OSG enrolled in the KSY scheme at 44 179 ICDS centres, were being reached by the ICDS sectors through the Adolescent Girls Scheme.

Figure 4: Adolescent Girls Anemia Control Programme - coverage and compliance of girls enrolled in school

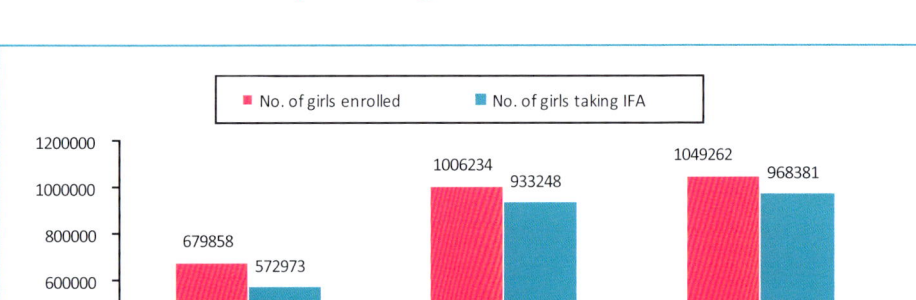

2.2 Lessons learnt

- Reaching school-going adolescent girls with WIFS through a joint effort of the education and health sectors is very effective. It is crucial to define the roles and responsibilities of each sector. The support of parents and teachers is critical.
- Reaching out-of-school girls (OSG) is a challenge and innovative approaches are required. Creating links with adolescent development programmes and non-government organizations could be experimented with.
- A fixed-day approach facilitates management of a WIFS programme.
- To ensure a regular supply of IFA supplements, a well-planned logistical system is essential.
- Involving district authorities from the Departments of Health and Education, associations of teachers and professional medical bodies right from the planning stage is helpful in creating a positive, supportive environment.
- Over 85% compliance with WIFS is feasible for adolescent girls in school or out of school with an effective communication and monitoring strategy. "Forgetfulness" is often the cause of poor compliance.
- Side-effects tend to decline when IFA supplements are consumed after food. However, since consumption of iron close to a meal reduces iron absorption, the best option is to take the supplements at least two hours after a meal, before retiring at night. It is critical to build this advice into the programme strategy.
- Over 50% of girls reported benefits from WIFS; those benefits should be promoted actively through the IEC strategy.
- Training programmes should stress skill-training in management of supply logistics, use of IEC materials and monitoring, rather than technical details.
- The use of individual monitoring cards aids, not only monitoring, but also compliance by helping to overcome the "forgetfulness" issue, which is noted to be the major factor responsible for non-compliance.
- The use of simple class and school registers, with information on each girl, facilitates effective monitoring of progress and is a useful tool for facilitating timely action.
- The WIFS programme is cost-effective; the cost per girl is only US$0.15.

References

1. Kotecha PV, *et al. Impact evaluation of adolescent girl's anaemia reduction programme*, Vadodara district. Government of Gujarat and UNICEF, 2002.
2. Gaonkar N. UNICEF Gandhinagar field office report (2008).
3. Karkar P. Personal communication, Ex–project Assistant, Adolescent Anaemia Reduction Programme, Department of Preventive and Social Medicine, Medical College Vadodara and Nutrition Consultant, July 2009.

2.3 Gujarat (India) WIFS Programme – A summary

Time framework and coverage	Age group	Anaemia prevalence	Intervention package	Nodal implementing agencies	Impact	Current status
• Pilot project – June 2001-Dec 2004. One district, 410 schools (VIII – IX std), 65 000 schoolgirls, 9536 OSG*. • Scaled up 2005 onwards, all 25 districts of the state. Estimated 1 million adolescent schoolgirls and 265 475 OSG covered.	• 12–19 years • 14–18 years	74.7% girls anaemic. 50% with low iron stores.	• WIFS • Nutrition education to improve dietary practices.	• Health Department • Education Department of the State Government	• Anaemia prevalence decreased from 74.7% to 53.2% in one year – 28.8% decrease. • Proportion of girls with normal iron levels increased from 25.3% to 46.8%. • Severe anaemia decreased from 1.6% to 0.5% (68% decrease).	State Government (Health and Education) covers over 1 million senior-school adolescent girls aged 14-18 years with WIFS in the entire state every Wednesday. Cost borne by the State Government. OSGs covered under the ICDS programme: 19% of OSG registered, with 44 179 ICDS centres covered.

Supply and consumption of WIFS

Composition, packaging and supply procurement	Cost	Specific approach used	Specific consumption instructions	IFA Supply to recipients		Supervision during WIFS consumption
				Free / purchased	Access	
• Each IFA tablet - 100 mg of elemental iron, 0.5 mg of folic acid. • Tablet identical to that used for pregnant women. • IFA supply from UNICEF to Health Department in the pilot phase. • IFA supply responsibilities in the scale-up phase shifted to Government.	• US$0.15 / girl / year (including cost of IFA, monitoring and brochure)	• Fixed-day (Wednesday) approach for both SG and OSG. Wednesday is not commonly a day of religious fasting and therefore selected. • In summer vacation, consumption advised at home.	• Consume after food since side-effects noted when consumed on an empty stomach.	• Free of cost to SG and OSG.	• For SG girls: schoolteachers under the Education Department. • For OSG: SG girls hand out IFA supply to OSG. • In urban areas, Integrated Child Development Service (ICDS) workers hand out the supply.	• Teachers in school • Not well defined • ICDS workers

* SG = School-going (girls)   OSG = Out-of-school girls

Efforts to increase compliance (IEC / Social mobilization / Strategy)

Positive attributes / benefits experienced	Side-effects reported and managed	Supplement-promotion strategy	Compliance
• 50.7% girls expressed benefits • increased work capacity • blood improved – redder • improved health • decreased pallor.	• Initially side-effects were reported by 29.7% of SG. In one year, side-effects reduced to 14.3%. Side-effects reported were abdominal pain, vomiting, giddiness and nausea. • Advised not to take WIFS on an empty stomach.	• School-level activities – slogan, drawing and debate competitions. • IEC materials – Brochure for girls (one / girl). Poster (2 sets / school) and a booklet on "20 frequently asked questions" to each school. • Monthly magazine for teachers.	• Compliance 89% in SG and 94% in OS girls. • During summer vacation, compliance reduced to 72.1% since girls advised to consume at home. Most common reason for poor compliance was forgetfulness (16.3% girls).

Training and monitoring

Training	Monitoring Individual cards / registers etc	Other positive contributing factors
• Training of teachers – importance of anaemia, skills in imparting nutrition education and monitoring.	• Monitoring at four levels – individual, class, school and cluster. • Individual level – simple "self-compliance card". • Class, school – registers.	• High-profile launch • Political system • Involvement of professional body (Indian Medical Association) and association (Teachers Association)

3. India (Madhya Pradesh)

3.1 Adolescent Anaemia Control Programme in two districts

	PROJECT AT A GLANCE
Date of programme	• Phase 1 – August 2002 – 2003 • Phase 2 - August 2003 – June 2008
Location	• Madhya Pradesh (India)
Number of participants	• Estimated 50 637 adolescent girls
Project managed by	• Integrated Child Health Services (ICDS), Health and Education Departments
Reduction in anaemia rate	• 8.9% in a 16-month period
Compliance rate	• 92%
Programme costs	• Cost of WIFS programme = US$0.33 per adolescent girl/year • Cost of WIFS = US$0.12 per adolescent girl/year

A. Project design

Background

In the state of Madhya Pradesh, in central India, a WIFS pilot project was implemented in two districts, Shivpuri and Guna, prior to scaling the project up throughout the state. This case study of Madhya Pradesh focuses on the implementation in these two districts from August 2002. More than 25 000 adolescent girls aged 10-18 years from the two districts were reached with a package of interventions comprising WIFS, health and nutrition education and biannual deworming. To reach adolescent girls in school and out of school, a seven-year (August 2002-2009) project plan was developed in consultation with partners from three primary sectors: Integrated Child Health Services (ICDS), Education and Health. The project was launched by the Minister of Social Welfare in a special function in the presence of senior district and block officials from all three sectors.

> More than 25 000 adolescent girls aged 10-18 years from these two districts were reached with a package of interventions comprising WIFS, nutrition education and biannual deworming.

Project goals

The objectives of the project were:

- To reduce anaemia prevalence in adolescent girls attending school by 50% by the end of the seven-year project period.
- For the State Government to adopt the project strategy for replication and extend it to girls out of school.
- For 70% of adolescent girls (10-19 yrs.) out of school to receive WIFS.
- To identify and strengthen at least one institution with regard to its capacity to provide technical support.
- To improve the dietary practices observed in at least 25% of adolescent girls by the end of seven years.

Monitoring

To facilitate monitoring, simple registers were developed. ICDS workers maintained a supply and compliance register for out-of-school girls, while teachers had the responsibility of maintaining records of IFA supply, consumption and compliance for girls attending school. A block-level task force, consisting of officials from all three sectors, reviewed the compiled monitoring reports and the project's progress every month. A district-level review was carried out at six-monthly intervals by the District Task Force, which had representatation from all three sectors.

B. Process and progress

IFA supply

The supplements used were identical to those used for pregnant women under the National Anaemia Control Programme. The non-sugar-coated IFA tablets were reddish-brown in colour and were blister-packed, with 10 tablets in each blister. Each IFA tablet contained 100 mg of elemental iron and 0.5 mg of folic acid.

IFA tablets were supplied by UNICEF to the ICDS, who then distributed the supply to block officials of the ICDS and the Education Department. The Education Block Official distributed the supply of IFA tablets at a monthly meeting of school officials. Likewise, a nodal block official or Child Development Project Officer distributed the supply to village-based ICDS centres, through the existing ICDS supply system, to reach girls not in school. The health sector was not involved in the supply logistics.

> **The rationale for selecting a common fixed day for both WIFS and immunization was that front-line health workers would be available at least once a month in a village/community to provide support for the WIFS programme.**

IFA supplements were provided to girls in school or out of school free of cost. In schools, IFA supplements were distributed and consumed by girls under the supervision of teachers on a fixed day. At the district level, the specific day that was selected for WIFS consumption was also the day designated as the fixed monthly immunization day. For example, all adolescent girls of the entire Guna district received IFA tablets every Tuesday, while immunization was held once a month, also on a Tuesday, in a specific village/community group. The latter was dependent on the visit plan of a health worker for routine immunization. Similarly, in Shivpuri district, the day designated for both WIFS and immunization was Saturday. The rationale for selecting a common fixed day for both WIFS and immunization was that front-line health workers would be available at least once a month in a village /community to provide support for the WIFS programme. The role of the health worker was limited to providing support by clarifying any queries related to anaemia or the use of WIFS. The involvement of the health sector in monthly sessions was encouraged, since it motivated adolescent girls to consume WIFS and helped in the organization of biannual deworming sessions. Deworming tablets (albendazole 400mg) were administered biannually to adolescent girls, linked to a vitamin A supplementation programme for less than five years.

On the fixed WIFS day, the first period of school, immediately after assembly, was used for the two primary project activities — health and nutrition education, and WIFS. To reach adolescent girls who were not in school, the project was linked to the ICDS network with the *Anganwadi* workers (AWW), one AWW per 1000 population being in charge of distributing IFA tablets, as well as supervising and monitoring consumption on the fixed day. On the fixed WIFS day, the out-of-school girls were mobilized and gathered together at a designated place, often next to a source of water, and provided with an IFA tablet by the AWW with the help of five to six adolescent girls. In addition, ICDS workers imparted health and nutrition education. In some ICDS centres, under the Adolescent Girls Scheme, known as *Kishori Shakti Yojna* (KSY), clubs of adolescent girls were formed with the objective of involving them in the management of the WIFS programme under the supervision of an ICDS worker.

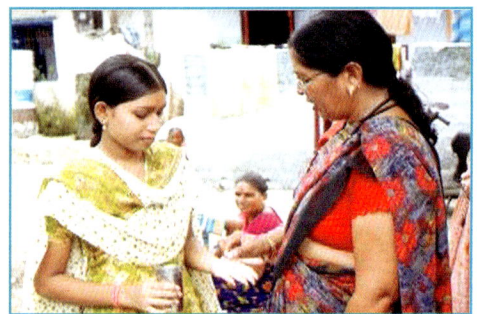 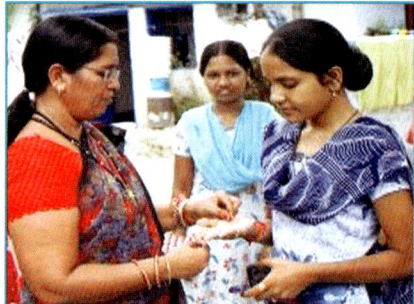

Provision of IFA Supplement by an *Anganwadi* Worker

Training

Training on the prevention of IDA through diet and WIFS, as well as the signs, symptoms and consequences of anaemia, was provided to programme workers from all three sectors (ICDS, education and health). Even though the health sector was not directly involved in implementing the WIFS programme, it was considered important to train health workers to ensure a uniform message on anaemia and the programme was imparted. Training manuals and booklets on frequently asked questions were developed for ICDS supervisors and schoolteachers. In addition, brochures were provided for Anganwadi workers, teachers, ICDS supervisors and community leaders to reinforce the information given at the training sessions. State directives issued by the State Government for the WIFS project were also shared at the training sessions at district and block levels.

Compliance

To reduce side-effects and improve compliance, girls were advised to consume the IFA supplement after a meal and not on an empty stomach. Additionally, the adolescent girls were advised to avoid drinking tea/coffee one to two hours prior to or after consumption of the supplements, so as not to inhibit iron absorption. The girls were advised to swallow IFA tablets using safe drinking water.

Teachers provided counselling for adolescent girls in schools to create demand and ensure high levels of compliance. For girls not in school, AWW and ICDS supervisors organized regular discussions. Discussion of positive experiences was found to be an effective strategy for improving compliance. Simple examples, such as:

> *"Laxmi in the peer group is stronger now. She takes an IFA supplement every week. She can carry 5-6 pots of water from the hand pump site. Laxmi was initially weak and carried only 2-3 pots of water at a time."*

were very motivating for the girls.

IEC activities

After a year of implementation, an evaluation was conducted and IEC activities were intensified as a result. Locally selected adolescent girls were used to impart information, ICDS workers were trained in counselling and an environment for increasing demand for WIFS was created through activities such as: slogan-writing, poetry competitions, skits and poster-making. In addition, appropriate messages in the form of slogans were written on the walls of schools and ICDS centres. ICDS workers were also involved in convincing community leaders and parents of adolescent girls of the importance of preventing iron and folic acid deficiency and the serious consequences of anaemia for school performance, work output and overall health. District extenders were appointed in each of the two districts to provide support for ICDS and education workers.

Evaluation

The impact of the project on anaemia and nutritional status, as well as on knowledge, attitudes and practice regarding anaemia, adolescent health and dietary practices, was studied by conducting a baseline and an impact study in OSG following 16 months of project implementation. The findings revealed that 94.5% girls had accepted the advice of routinely consuming IFA tablets. Compliance was very high, with 92.8% girls consuming over 50-100 IFA tablets in a 16-month intervention period; 3.5% of rural girls and 1.8% of urban girls consumed less than 25 tablets in the same period. For all but 16.1% of girls, an ICDS worker, a mother, a family member, or a friend supervised the consumption of WIFS.

Another study was undertaken of 1473 girls. Of these, 1392 reported that they had consumed IFA tablets. Side-effects had been experienced by only 74 of these 1392 girls (5.3%). However, with periodic counselling built into the programme, the majority of girls who reported side-effects (77% of the 74 with side-effects) had continued taking the IFA supplements. In addition, 86% of girls believed WIFS to be beneficial, while 31% had experienced benefits such as decreased fatigue, increased energy, reduced illness and dizziness, improved appetite and a general sense of well-being. These benefits were highlighted in the counselling sessions.

> **86% of girls believed WIFS to be beneficial, while 31% experienced benefits such as decreased fatigue, increased energy, reduced illness and dizziness, improved appetite and a general sense of well-being. These benefits were highlighted in the counselling sessions.**

Table 8: Girls consuming WIFS and side-effects experienced		
	Number	%
Girls taking WIFS	1392	94.5*
Girls with side-effects	74	5.3
- Nausea / vomiting	25	1.7
- Constipation	8	0.5
- Diarrhoea	5	0.3
- Black stools	4	0.3
- Abdominal pain	8	0.5
- Heartburn	2	0.1
- Headache	1	0.1
- Dizziness	21	1.4
Girls with side-effects (74)		
- continued with IFA	57	77.0
- discontinued with IFA	17	23.0

* Total girls studied = 1473

The study revealed that, following one year of supplementation, the percentage of girls with anaemia had decreased significantly from 87.8% to 80%. Over one third had moderate anaemia at baseline, while only 1.6% had severe anaemia. The impact data (Figure 5) indicates that there was a significant positive shift in haemoglobin levels, with a 36.6% reduction in moderate anaemia cases and an increase of 8.9% in cases of mild anaemia. The overall reduction of anaemia therefore, while significant, remained low, at about 8.9%, despite high coverage and compliance rates. It appears that a higher reduction in the overall anaemia prevalence rate will require additional months of WIFS consumption, since almost 60 % of girls were mildly anaemic at the end of the year. The findings indicate that, in situations where the anaemia prevalence rate is over 80%, with over 50% of those cases being moderately anaemic, the shift to a normal haemoglobin range may take longer using WIFS. However, a WIFS programme is sustainable and has benefits that encourage compliance. Furthermore, WIFS has a low incidence of side-effects.

Figure 5: Prevalence of anaemia among the girls studied at baseline and after one year of supplements

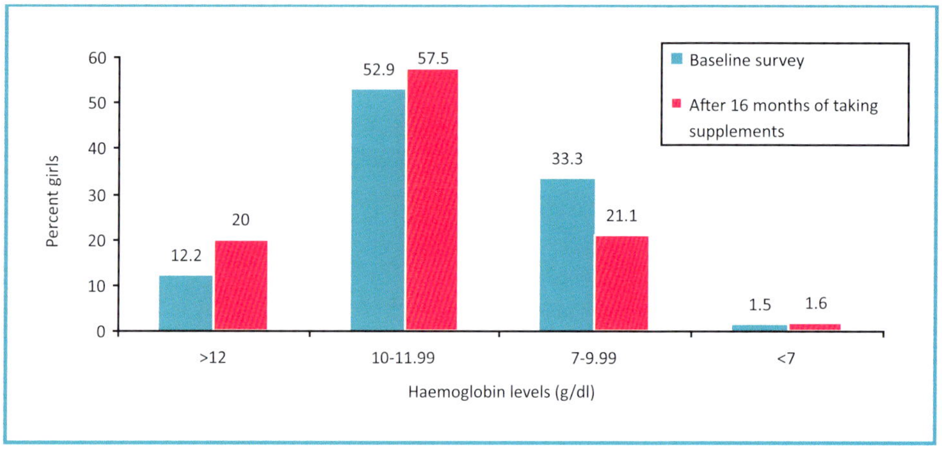

Cost

The cost per adolescent girl was studied for one of the project districts, Shivpuri, where 70 272 girls were reached with WIFS. The cost per adolescent girl per year was assessed to be about US$0.33. The cost estimate includes the cost of IFA tablets and the additional costs of communication, training and monitoring activities. Due to the low cost of introducing WIFS through the education and ICDS systems, the State Government has developed a plan of action for introducing WIFS in the ICDS Adolescent Girls Scheme, as well as in the Adolescent Health Programme of the NRHM.

3.2 Lessons learnt

- Consumption of WIFS is cost-effective and resulted in positive shifts in haemoglobin levels in adolescent girls in a period of 16 months. The annual cost per girl is about US$0.33.
- A WIFS Programme should not be limited to WIFS alone, but should be part of a more comprehensive programme, including health and nutrition education and biannual provision of deworming.

- A fixed-day strategy is effective for reaching adolescent girls both in and out of schools with WIFS. In selecting the fixed day, if the same day as the immunization day is chosen, it will ensure the availability of a health worker for the WIFS programme at least once a month and increase the possibility of support from health workers in a programme managed by a non-health sector.

- Reaching girls out of school is a challenge. However, forming adolescent clubs and involving these girls in implementation of the WIFS programme facilitates overall management.

- Higher compliance can be achieved by avoiding consumption of IFA supplements on an empty stomach. Moreover, this advice, combined with effective counselling, improves compliance.

- Sharing of positive experiences and stressing the reported benefits of IFA supplements contributes to increasing demand for the supplements and high compliance.

- Use of simple monitoring registers to record IFA supply, consumption and compliance is useful for recording and analysing progress, as well as highlighting potential problems.

- A WIFS programme can be successfully implemented by non-health sectors, but it is critical that the health sector is still involved so that technical issues can be resolved. Involvement of the health sector will also influence the community to be more accepting of the programme and will aid in creating a more supportive environment.

- The reduction in the anaemia rate, in this project, was only about 8.9% after 16 months of WIFS supplementation, despite high coverage and compliance rates. However, during that period there was a much greater reduction in cases of moderate anaemia (36%). At the end of one year, almost 60% of girls were found to be mildly anaemic. Other causes of anaemia need to be explored; daily iron/folic acid supplements may be needed and/or other measures to address other causes of anaemia.

References

1. Sharma K, Gandhi H. *A study on assessing the impact of adolescent anaemia control project among out of school adolescent girls, a midterm evaluation in Shivpuri district, Madhya Pradesh.* Department of Women and Child Development, State Government of Madhya Pradesh, India and UNICEF.

2. Agarwal V. Personal communication UNICEF Bhopal field office report (2008).

3.3 Madhya Pradesh (India) WIFS Programme – A summary

Time framework and coverage	Age group	Anaemia prevalence	Intervention package	Nodal implementing agencies	Impact	Current status
Phase 1 – pilot August 2002 – August 2003 • 1 district (8 blocks) 25 000 girls Phase 2 – scaled up August 2003 – June 2008 • All 13 blocks of two districts • 25 637 girls	10-18 years SG* and OSG* girls	87.8% of adolescent girls anaemic. Severe anaemia only 1.6%.	- IFA (WIFS) - Deworming (biannual) - Family-life education, including anaemia prevention and dietary iron.	• Health • Education • ICDS	• Anaemia prevalence decreased significantly from 87.8% to 80% in 16 months – a significant decrease of 8.9%.	WIFS being incorporated into the State Implementation Plan of National Rural Health Mission (NRHM) for SG. For OSG, statewide implementation through ICDS.

Supply and consumption of WIFS

Composition, packaging and supply procurement	Cost	Specific approach used	Specific consumption instructions	IFA Supply to recipients		Supervision during WIFS consumption
				Free / purchased	Access	
100 mg of elemental iron + 0.5 mg of folic acid tablets, non-sugar-coated, brown-red, blister packs of 10-30. Supplied by UNICEF.	US$ 0.33/adolescent girl /year. Cost of IFA supplement = US$ 0.12/year for 52 tablets.	Fixed-day varies in two districts (Tuesday and Saturday), same as immunization day once a month.	• Consume IFA after meal and not on empty stomach. • Avoid drinking tea / coffee one hour prior to or after consumption of WIFS. • Use safe drinking water.	WIFS free of cost to adolescent girls.	• OSG by ICDS worker. OSG mobilized and collected in a group next to a source of water. • SG by teacher in the first period of the fixed day.	OSG supervised by the front-line worker (Anganwadi worker) of the ICDS programme and mother, family or friends. For SGs, nodal teachers supervised.

* SG = School-going (girls) OSG = Out-of-school girls

Efforts to increase compliance (IEC / Social mobilization / Strategy)

Positive attributes / benefits experienced	Side-effects reported and managed	Supplement-promotion strategy	Compliance
Benefits of WIFS were perceived by 86% of the 1392 girls who were consuming IFA supplements, and 31% experienced benefits such as - lowering of fatigue; - increase in energy; - reduction in dizziness, illness; - improved appetite; - feeling better.	Side-effects were experienced by 5.3% of the 1392 girls followed up, such as headache, vomiting / nausea, constipation, diarrhoea, black stools, dizziness.	• Create an environment for increasing demand – slogan-writing, poetry competition, skits, poster-making, catchy slogans (schools + ICDS walls). • Convince community leaders and parents. • Share positive experiences. • Conduct regular counselling of girls at community gatherings at the village level. • Share positive experiences with one another in group. • IEC materials, including folders, posters, etc. • Wall-writing in villages by schoolchildren and at Anganwadi Centre by OSG.	• Compliance – 92%. • Regular sharing of benefits helped in increasing compliance.

Training and monitoring

Training	Monitoring Individual cards / registers etc	Other positive contributing factors
Training – ICDS workers, teachers and district officers of ICDS, education and health sector. Health sector officers were trainers. Focus of training • Causes, signs and symptoms of iron deficiency and anaemia. • Prevention and treatment of anaemia – WIFS and dietary measures. • Counselling skills for imparting uniform message and information, and social mobilization of teachers. • Prevention of iron deficiency – dietary measures and supplements. • Operationalization of state directives on WIFS. Special manual • Training manual developed for teachers and ICDS supervisor. • IEC – FAQs, booklets, brochures.	• OSG – Simple supply and compliance monitoring registers maintained by ICDS workers. • For schoolgirls – register for recording consumption – IFA supply register for each school. • Block review meeting every month. • District review every six months.	• Programme extenders specifically appointed in each district. • Health sector involved on immunization day to motivate adolescent girls.

4. India (Uttar Pradesh)

4.1 Weekly iron and folic acid supplementation along with counselling among school-going and out-of-school girls

PROJECT AT A GLANCE	
Date of programme	• Phase 1 – September 2001 – December 2002 • Phase 2 - January 2003 – December 2004 • Phase 3 – January 2005 – December 2006
Location	• Uttar Pradesh (India)
Number of participants	• Estimated 150 700 adolescent girls
Project managed by	• NGO in collaboration with Health and Education Departments and Integrated Child Health Services (ICDS)
Reduction in anaemia rate	• 46.8% in a one-year period
Compliance rate	• 90% in SG • 86% in OSG
Programme costs	• Cost of WIFS programme = US$0.36 per adolescent girl/year • Cost of WIFS = US$0.12 per adolescent girl/year

A. Project design

Background

In 1998, the Government of India recommended that large-scale demonstration projects should be undertaken to study the feasibility and effectiveness of WIFS in addressing the problem of anaemia in adolescent girls. Accordingly, a district-level project for adolescent girls, both in and out of school, was planned for one of the 70 districts of Uttar Pradesh state.

Uttar Pradesh is a northern Indian state with a total population of 180 million, 20 million of them adolescents. The objective of the district-level project was to integrate an implementation strategy with other ongoing development programmes to reduce anaemia in adolescent girls aged 10 to 19 years. The project intervention consisted of WIFS, six-monthly deworming and family-life education.

Target group

A comprehensive project entitled UMANG[9] (Uplifting Marriage Age, Nutrition, and Growth) was launched in Lucknow, a central district of Uttar Pradesh. The district has 10 administrative rural and urban blocks, with a population of 3 647 834. The project was launched in three phases. Phase 1 was conducted from September 2001 to December 2002 in one administrative block among girls aged 11 to 18 years who were not in school (OSG). Phase 2 was conducted from January 2003 to December 2004 in two administrative blocks also among girls aged 11 to 18 years, but including both schoolgirls (SG) and OSG. Phase 3 was conducted from January 2005 to December 2006 in all 10 administrative blocks of the district among SG and OSG aged 10 to 19 years (Table 9). Between September 2001 and December 2006, one third of adolescent girls, a total of 150 700 girls (73 700 OSG and 77 000 SG), were covered.

---

9   The acronym UMANG means "joy with an element of hope" in the local language.

Table 9: Coverage of OSG and SG in one district					
Phase	No. of blocks (total population)	Age group (yr)	No. of ICDS centres[a]	No. of schools	Girls covered
Phase 1 - Sep 2001– Dec 2002	1 (85 383)	11–18	95	–	3800 OSG
Phase 2 - Jan 2003–Dec 2004	2 (324 087)	11–18	265[b]	100	22 695 (12 695 OSG and 10 000 SG)
Phase 3 - Jan 2005–Dec 2006	10 in rural and urban areas (3 047 854)	10–19	1275	351	150 700 (73 700 OSG and 77 000 SG

a. ICDS (Integrated Child Development Services) centres are established by the government for each population of about 1000.
b. There were 95 centres in one block and 170 in the other.

Programme roles and responsibility for OSG

A state-based NGO supported implementation of the UMANG project in coordination with three primary government agencies: Health, Education, and Integrated Child Development Services (ICDS). The elected rural development representatives, who were members of Panchayati Raj institutions, the grassroots units of self-government, were fully involved.

Phase 1 of the project targeted OSG and was built on to the Reproductive Child Health Programme, part of the Primary Health and Family Welfare Services, and the ongoing Adolescent Girls Scheme (ADS) of the ICDS. Under ADS, only three adolescent girls from the most deprived section of the community are selected from a population of about 1000. Under the UMANG project, these three ADS girls were trained to mobilize and form a group of 20 to 25 adolescent girls, referred to as the "UMANG group". These girls were also trained to provide support to ICDS workers in keeping records of IFA supplies and in recording compliance. The UMANG group members, using a girl-to-girl approach, often reached an additional 20 to 50 girls in the community who did not directly participate in the regular UMANG group meetings.

Monitoring

For OSG, the monitoring system was limited to the UMANG leaders recording the supply of IFA tablets and their consumption in a register at the ICDS centre. Since consumption was not supervised, the record was based on the reports of adolescent girls to the group leader. However, records were not routinely completed.

For SG, compliance was recorded on individual cards by the girls themselves and this information was then transferred to class registers by nodal teachers. The data compiled at school level was shared every month with the nodal NGO. Compliance records were reviewed periodically by teachers and the nodal NGO.

Annual WIFS monitoring card

Details of class / school monitoring register

B. Process and progress

IFA supply

The intervention for all SG and OSG consisted of WIFS, deworming tablets given at six-monthly intervals, and family-life education. UNICEF and the State Government of Uttar Pradesh supplied both IFA and albendazole. The red, non-sugar-coated IFA tablets contained 100 mg of elemental iron and 0.5mg of folic acid. The composition of the tablets was identical to that of tablets prescribed for daily consumption by pregnant women under the National Anaemia Control Programme of the Government of India. Tetanus toxoid injections, supplied by the State Government, were also administered to some girls by the Health Department.

The fourth Saturday of the month became the fixed day for UMANG meetings for OSG. Each girl in the UMANG group was provided with four or five IFA tablets per month from a blister pack of 10 or 30 tablets for her own consumption and an additional four or eight IFA tablets for reaching one or two girls in the community. Deworming tablets (albendazole, 400 mg) were administered to OSG along with the first dose of IFA and at six-monthly intervals thereafter. The consumption of IFA tablets by the OSG group was not supervised.

> The intervention for all SG and OSG consisted of WIFS, deworming tablets at six-monthly intervals, and family-life education.

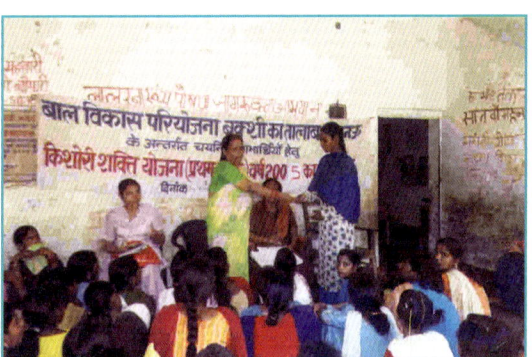

Distribution of IFA tablets to out-of-school girls (OSG)

A fixed day of the week (Saturday) was also designated as UMANG Day for SG. Saturday was selected as WIFS Day since on this day it was compulsory, in senior and middle schools, to hold classes on the subject of "Socially useful activities". IFA tablets were provided and consumed by most of the girls under the direct supervision of teachers and class monitors. However, a few girls who complained of gastrointestinal problems were advised to consume the tablets after dinner and were therefore not supervised. Deworming tablets were administered every six months, in February and August.

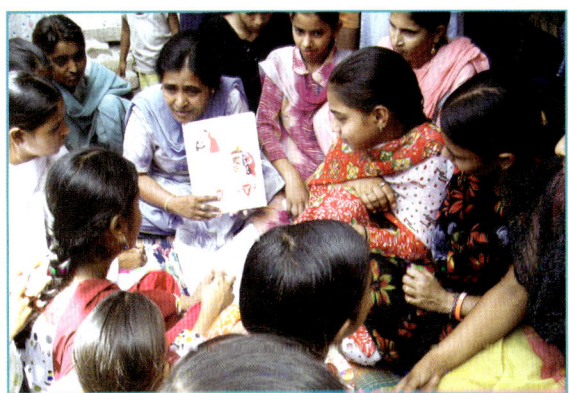

Family life education session

IEC activities and training

Family-life education was provided to OSG by ICDS Anganwadi workers, with the support of NGOs. The benefits of regular consumption of IFA tablets and the importance of adhering to the weekly dose were discussed. Special emphasis was placed on relating the consumption of IFA to increasing energy levels for daily work, reducing lethargy, increasing concentration at work, improving skin appearance/glow and regularizing menstruation. To prevent adverse effects, such as abdominal pain, nausea, or other gastrointestinal problems, the girls were advised to consume the tablets after dinner or the last large meal of the day before going to sleep.

The purpose of family-life education sessions was to:

- provide education on values;
- encourage positive thinking;
- discuss the physical and psychological changes that occur throughout adolescence;
- provide health and nutrition information, including details on the importance of WIFS;
- educate girls regarding the right age for marriage and conception; and
- provide information about sexually transmitted diseases, including HIV/AIDS.

The sessions focused on a different theme each month. The topics varied from development and care during adolescence to young child and family care. To encourage girls to participate in the sessions, they were asked to write questions (which they were often not comfortable asking in the presence of peers) on pieces of paper and put them in a question box to be discussed in the sessions.

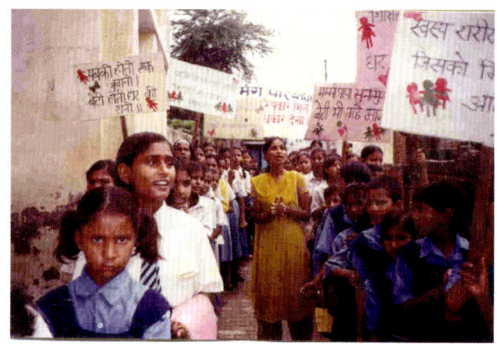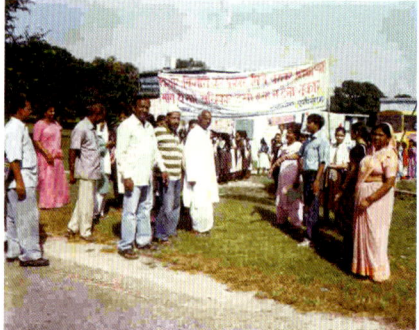

School rally for community mobilization

For SG, the intervention package was introduced through the school system. The middle and senior schools of a district, enrolling girls aged 10 to 19 years, were mapped. A designated NGO trained two teachers per school, using a specific training manual developed for the project. Posters with culturally relevant information were provided for each classroom.

Family-life education sessions for SG were held twice a month on Saturdays, as described for the OSG group. Information materials consisted of an illustrated training manual for the teachers and posters for the classrooms.

Evaluation

In the first phase, 3800 OSG attached to 95 ICDS centres were covered. A baseline survey and a six-month post-supplementation study on knowledge, attitudes and practices were conducted. The findings (Table 10) revealed that the family-life education sessions resulted in a significant increase in awareness of anaemia and knowledge of preventive measures, especially the role of IFA tablets.

> The family-life education sessions resulted in a significant increase in awareness of anaemia and knowledge of preventive measures, especially the role of IFA tablets.

Table 10: Knowledge of anaemia among OSG at baseline and after six months of family-life education (percentage of girls)

Type of knowledge	Age 11–14 yr		Age 15–18 yr	
	Baseline	After six months	Baseline	After six months
Awareness of anaemia	44.0	94.7[a]	64.1	98.9[b]
Preventive measures				
- IFA tablets	4.2	38.0	10.3	37.3
- Improved diet	12.5	16.8	21.8	31.4
- Both diet and tablets	1.5	35.3	3.6	22.8
- Medicines and tonics	26.0	6.5	27.9	4.6
- Other	0.8	0.5	1.2	0.3
- DNK (do not know)	56.6	7.3	39.1	4.4

a. $t = 11.026$ ($p < .01$).
b. $t = 8.244$ ($p < .01$).

After six months of WIFS, the mean haemoglobin value in OSG improved significantly, from 110 to 118 g/L (t = 6.234, p < .01), and the percentage of girls with anaemia (haemoglobin < 120 g/L) decreased from 55.0% to 39.8% (Figure 6). The prevalence of severe anaemia (haemoglobin < 70 g/L) decreased from 2.3% to 1.0%, the prevalence of moderate anaemia (haemoglobin 70 to 99 g/L) from 15.3% to 4.9%, and the prevalence of mild anaemia (haemoglobin 100 to 119 g/L) from 37.4% to 33.9%. Twelve months of intervention resulted in further improvement in haemoglobin levels and a reduction in the prevalence of anaemia (Figure 6).

Figure 6: Haemoglobin levels in OSG after six and 12 months of WIFS. Haemoglobin levels ≥ 120 g/L indicate no anaemia, < 70 g/L severe anaemia, 70 to 99 g/L moderate anaemia, and 100 to 119 g/L mild anaemia.

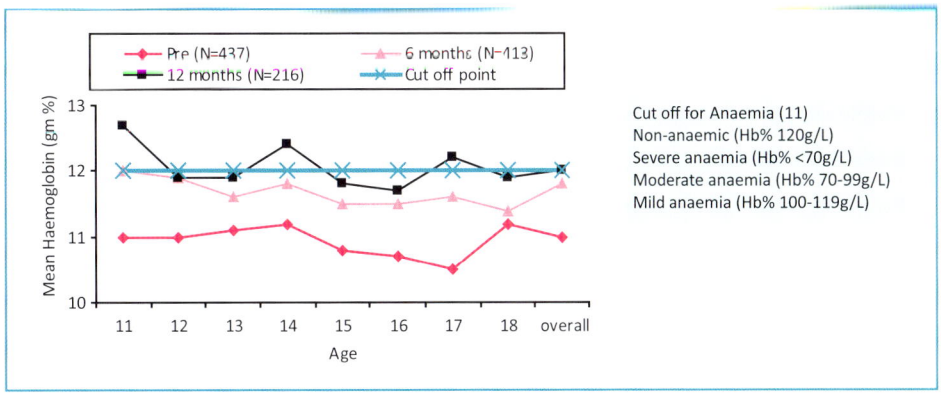

Haemoglobin levels were also measured in SG selected at random from both blocks of Phase 2. Figure 7 presents the change in anaemia status at six months. The mean haemoglobin levels improved in SG from 108 to 118 g/L (t = 9.756, p < .01) and the anaemia prevalence rate decreased from 73.8% to 46.3% (t = 7.378, p < .01)

Figure 7: Anaemia status of schoolgirls after six months of WIFS. Haemoglobin levels < 120 g/L indicate anaemia, < 70 g/L severe anaemia, 70 to 99 g/L moderate anaemia, 100 to 119 g/L mild anaemia and ≥ 120 g/L no anaemia.

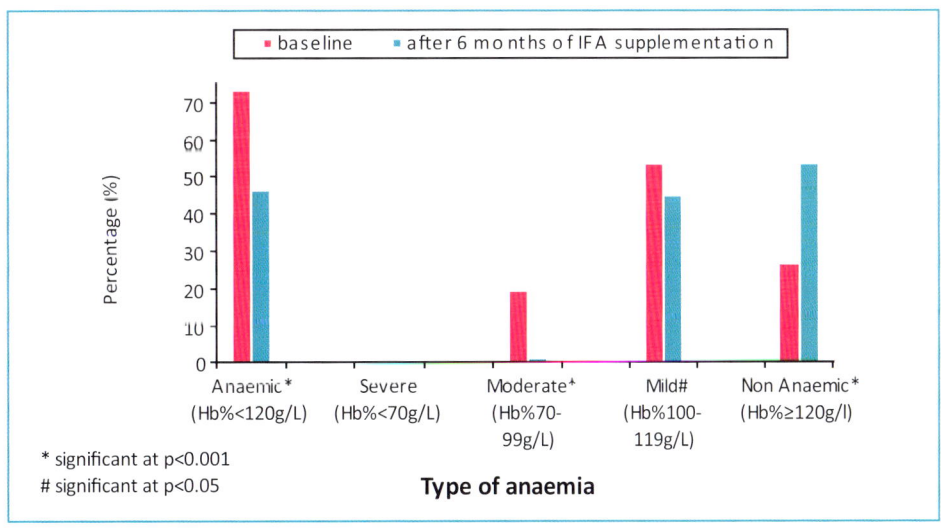

The effectiveness of WIFS in reducing anaemia was studied in SG and OSG selected at random in 2003, 2004 and 2006. In 2003, only 26.7% of girls were non-anaemic.

After four years, the percentage of girls who were non-anaemic had increased remarkably to 74.6 % (Table 11). Reluctance to be pricked for blood samples was a major constraint of the study.

| Table 11: Anaemia status of combined OSG and SG in 2003, 2004 and 2006 ||||||
| Year | Number | Total | Anaemic (haemoglobin < 120 g/L) ||| Non-anaemic (haemoglobin > 120 g/L) |
			Severe (haemoglobin < 70g/L)	Moderate (haemoglobin 70–99g/L)	Mild (haemoglobin 100–119 g/L)	
2003	1173	73.3	0	7.9	65.4	26.7
2004	870	39.0	0	1.1	37.9	61.0
2006	301	25.4	1.6	6.5	17.3	74.6

Compliance

It is interesting to note that there was no significant difference in the effect of six months of supplementation on haemoglobin levels between supervised SG and unsupervised OSG. It was observed that holding regular education sessions and compiling information on compliance for IFA tablets every month played a more important role in increasing compliance than supervising consumption of IFA tablets.

Routine monitoring information is available only for SG and indicates that the compliance rate with weekly supplementation remained high in all three phases of implementation. During the first year, 2003, as well as in 2006, SG had a compliance rate of over 90%. The individual monitoring cards maintained by the girls, not only provided a record of compliance, but also served as a reminder for weekly consumption of the tablets.

Analysis of data from 150 randomly selected OSG after at least two years of intervention showed high compliance, with 86.0% of girls regularly consuming the tablets (Table 12). The primary reason for poor compliance was forgetfulness (52.4%), while 28.6% cited "health problems" as the reason. Around 83% consumed the tablets at least an hour after dinner, which may have contributed to the low percentage of girls with adverse effects. Almost all the girls (99.3%) drank only water while consuming the tablets.

A major factor responsible for the success of the large project was its motivational strategy. Despite poor monitoring of OSG, timely and repeated counselling, with an emphasis on the positive effects of WIFS, appears to have contributed to its

> It was observed that holding regular education sessions and compiling information on compliance for IFA tablets every month played a more important role in increasing compliance than supervising consumption of IFA tablets.

success. These findings confirm that, even in a large-scale weekly supplementation project, appropriate counselling can overcome poor compliance. A focus on the benefits of WIFS appears to be as effective as supervising consumption.

Table 12: Characteristics of consumption of IFA tablets by 150 OSG	
Characteristic	% (No.) of girls
Weekly consumption	
Yes	86.0 (129)
No	14.0 (21)
Reasons for not consuming	
Forgot	52.4 (11)
Health effects	28.6 (6)*
Other	19.0 (4)
Perceived impact of tablets	
Positive	62.7 (94)
Negative	18.7 (28)
None	18.7 (28)
Time of consumption	
Any time	16.7 (25)
After dinner	82.7 (124)
On an empty stomach	0.6 (1)
Manner of consumption	
With tea or coffee	0.7 (1)
With water	99.3 (149)

* 6 OSG (4 %) out of a total of 150 reported adverse effects on health

Cost

Cost per beneficiary was calculated and included the cost of IFA supplement, educational materials and activities, training and monitoring. In Phase 1, the annual cost was rather high at Rs 119.62 or about US$3 per beneficiary. The annual cost was reduced remarkably to Rs 14.60 (US$0.36) per beneficiary when the project implementation moved from the pilot phase in one block in 2001–2002 to covering the entire district in 2006 (Table 13). The district-level project demonstrated that the WIFS programme, as it was built on to existing programmes, cost only about one third of a dollar per beneficiary annually. Moreover, the cost was significantly reduced when the implementation shifted from an experimental project to a programme model and was linked to ongoing health or education programmes.

Table 13: Cost of the intervention			
Year	No. of beneficiaries	Yearly per capita cost (Rs)	Yearly per capita cost (US$)
2003	3800	119.62	2.96
2004	22 695	58.60	1.45
2006	150 700	14.60	0.36

From this study it was concluded that, in a developing country such as India, provision of WIFS to adolescent girls should be viewed as one of the most important nutrition interventions, since it increases work and school performance and reduces the risk of anaemia during pregnancy. The latter will significantly reduce rates of maternal mortality, fetal growth retardation, perinatal mortality and low birth-weight. WIFS for adolescent girls has been recognized as a critical component of the Reproductive and Child Health Programme and maternal and child nutrition, and has been included in the state plan on Adolescent Health under the National Rural Health Mission (NRHM). Since December 2008, the entire state of 71 districts has included the WIFS programme in the District Plan of Action and a total of 6500 middle schools (standard VI-VIII) are being covered in the first phase, with the State Government bearing the cost of implementation and IFA supplements.

4.2 Lessons learnt

- WIFS, combined with effective counselling, is a cost-effective intervention for the prevention of anaemia in adolescent girls in institutional and community settings.

- Reaching girls in schools with WIFS is a feasible, practical and low-cost strategy. Girls out of school can, to a great extent, be reached through forming groups of OSG and introducing a well-planned girl-to-girl approach.

- IFA tablets, like those used under the national programme for pregnant mothers for daily intake, are well accepted by adolescent girls as weekly supplements. Use of identical tablets for adolescents and pregnant mothers will facilitate logistical management.

- Demand for WIFS and a high degree of compliance can be achieved by emphasizing the positive benefits of WIFS through a comprehensive communication and motivation strategy.

- To sustain the interest of adolescent girls in education sessions, WIFS can be used as an entry point for educational activities. It is important not to limit the content of education sessions to iron nutrition or anaemia. Including topics that are important to adolescents, such as value education, positive thinking, the importance of the right age for marriage and conception, family care, etc. are more appealing to young growing girls and therefore important for sustaining interest. Fixing a specific theme for the month provides structure to the education sessions and helps maintain the interest of adolescent girls.

- A "question box" is a useful tool for encouraging girls to participate in group discussions.

- Monitoring can be done at three levels for SG — individual, class and school. At an individual level, simple compliance cards are helpful. Simple registers with information on each student are easy to maintain at a class or school level. Individual cards and registers are comparatively difficult to maintain for girls who are not enrolled in schools.

- The use of individual compliance cards, not only helps in self-monitoring, but also acts as a tool for reminding girls to adhere to the weekly schedule. The use of such cards increases compliance.

- In a large-scale WIFS programme, effective communication to accompany the distribution of IFA supplements is crucial. Timely and repeated counselling is effective in increasing WIFS compliance to over 90%, even in the absence of supervision. It is essential to emphasize the benefits of WIFS, such as increased energy levels for daily work, reduced lethargy, increased concentration at work and at school, enhanced glow and improved appearance of skin, and more regular menstruation.

- A fixed-day strategy facilitates, not only the distribution of WIFS, but overall programme implementation, including organizing education sessions and improving compliance.

- Poor compliance is mainly due to forgetfulness rather than side effects. Timely and repeated counselling helps increase compliance. Further use of a fixed-day strategy and establishing a habit of taking supplements at a particular time of day, such as after dinner or before going to bed, helps overcome forgetfulness and increase compliance.

- Adverse effects are reported by a small percentage of girls — less than 6%. It is important to inform adolescent girls of the possible side-effects of WIFS but, at the same time, caution must be taken not to overemphasize the side-effects.

- To reduce side-effects, it is critical to advise girls to take supplements before going to sleep, at least two hours after dinner, if possible, as this helps to increase iron absorption.

- Cost is significantly reduced when the programme is implemented on a large scale and built on to an ongoing education or women's health development programme.

- Advocacy with concerned health and non-health sectors for inclusion of WIFS interventions is crucial.

References

1. Vir SC, *et al*. Weekly iron and folic acid supplementation with counselling reduces anaemia in adolescent girls: A large effectiveness study in Uttar Pradesh, India. *Food and nutrition bulletin*, 29, 186-194(2008).

4.3 Uttar Pradesh (India) WIFS Programme – A summary

Time framework and coverage	Age group	Anaemia prevalence	Intervention package	Nodal implementing agencies	Impact	Current status
Phase 1: Sept 2001 – Dec 2002, one administrative block unit, only OSG* = 3800	11-18 years	73.3% of adolescent girls anaemic	• WIFS • Biannual deworming (400 mg albendazole) • Family-life education	• NGO, in collaboration with State Government / (Health Education and ICDS sectors).	• In the first 12 months, 46.8% decrease in anaemia prevalence, from 73.3% to 39.0%. • Anaemia prevalence decreased from 73.3% to 25.4% between 2003 and 2006.	• Provision of WIFS to adolescent schoolgirls included in the National Rural Health Mission (NRHM). • SG of 6500 schools (std VI to VIII) were covered in phase 1. • Under NRHM, since Dec 2008, the entire state (71 districts) has been covered. • OSG planned to be covered under the ICDS scheme.
Phase 2: Jan 2003 – Dec 2004, OSG + SG = 22, 695	11-18 years					
Phase 3: Jan 2005 – Dec 2006	10-19 years					
Total coverage in 2006 = 150 700 girls (includes 73 700 OSG*)						

Supply and consumption of WIFS

Composition, packaging and supply procurement	Cost	Specific approach used	Specific consumption instructions	IFA Supply to recipients		Supervision during WIFS consumption
				Free / purchased	Access	
UNICEF and State Government of Uttar Pradesh (UP) – IFA tablets contain 100 mg of elemental iron as ferrous sulphate and 0.5 mg of folic acid. Blister pack of 30 red, non-sugar-coated tablets, with each strip containing 10 tablets.	Cost = US $ 0.36 / girl / year. This includes cost of IFA supplement, training, IEC, monitoring. Cost of tablets US $ 0.12 / girl / year.	Fixed day – Saturday.	Advised to consume IFA after dinner or the last large meal of the day before going to sleep.	Free of cost to SG and OSG.	• Adolescent girls' group leaders under ICDS project handed IFA to OSG. Also girl-to-girl approach used. A blister pack of 8-10 tablets for monthly consumption was given to OSG for self-consumption and for handing over to another OSG. • In schools, teachers, helped by monitors, distributed tablets every week (Saturday).	• OSG – not supervised. • SG – consumed IFA under the direct supervision of teachers or class monitors.

* SG = School-going (girls)   OSG = Out-of-school girls

Efforts to increase compliance (IEC / Social mobilization / Strategy)

Positive attributes / benefits experienced	Side-effects reported and managed	Supplement-promotion strategy	Compliance
62.7% reported a positive experience following WIFS consumption.	18.7% reported side-effects, such as vomiting, nausea, diarrhoea and black stools.	IEC strategy on WIFS was part of overall family-life education, emphasising the importance of nutrition, iron-rich food and adhering to the weekly preventive IFA dose. The benefits of WIFS were routinely described. Special emphasis was placed on relating the consumption of IFA supplements to increasing energy levels for daily work, reduced lethargy, increasing concentration at work, improved school performance, improving skin glow and appearance, and regular menstruation. A question-box technique was introduced in schools. Family-life education was held twice a month.	Compliance 90% in SG and 86% in OSG. Primary reason for poor compliance – forgetfulness – reported by 52.4%.

Training and monitoring

Training	Monitoring — Individual cards / registers etc	Other positive contributing factors
• For SG – trained teachers of middle and senior schools of districts. • Training materials comprised a simple illustrated training manual for teachers, ICDS workers and adolescent girls' group leaders.	• For OSG – Register used for recording supply and weekly consumption. • For SG – individual cards and group registers.	• Timely repeated counselling on the benefits of WIFS during adolescence and in future during pregnancy.

5. Egypt

5.1 Adolescent Anaemia Prevention Programme in Egypt (Upper Egypt)

PROJECT AT A GLANCE	
Date of programme	• Phase 1 – September 1999 • Phase 2 – February 2000 • Phase 3 – 2001
Location	• Upper Egypt (Egypt)
Number of participants	• Since 2008, 6 000 000 boys and girls 10-20 have been covered
Project managed by	• Health Department, Ministry of Education, Social Health Insurance Programme
Reduction in anaemia rate	• 20% in a six-month period
Compliance rate	• 92.2% in Phase 1
Programme costs	• Data not available

A. Project design

Target group

Preliminary results from Egypt's Demographic and Health Survey, conducted in 2000, showed that 30% of adolescents were anaemic. Poor eating habits, with low consumption of iron-rich foods and high consumption of foods that inhibit iron absorption, such as tea and whole bread, were found to be factors contributing to poor iron status and anaemia. Adolescence was considered an opportune time to address anaemia since, during this period of life, ID has serious implications for growth as well as building of pre-pregnancy iron stores. Moreover, it was considered feasible to reach subjects through a school health programme, since 73% of the adolescent population at the age of 14 years was enrolled in secondary education. A school programme for students of 11-19 years in preparatory and secondary grades was therefore launched to reach both adolescent boys and girls for anaemia prevention.

Programme roles and responsibilities

The Government of Egypt developed a comprehensive and sustainable policy for youths, which targets about 13 million adolescents, and the Government's Health Insurance Organization (HIO) expanded the programme to cover all schoolchildren. HIO provides preventive and curative health services under its Social Health Insurance Programme (SHIP), which works in collaboration with the Department of Maternal and Child Health and the Ministry of Health and Population. With a high rate of anaemia in adolescents, SHIP implemented the Adolescent Anaemia Prevention Programme with the objective of reducing existing anaemia rates and preventing anaemia in preparatory and secondary schools. The United States Agency for International Development (USAID) collaborated with the Ministry of Health and Population's Healthy Mother/Healthy Child Project and SHIP to implement the programme.

The programme was launched by SHIP in five governorates in three phases to ensure that the operational issues for WIFS and nutrition education were addressed in the first two phases and any logistical problems or cultural issues could be resolved prior to scaling up the programme in the third phase. SHIP, whose headquarters in Cairo has district and governorate administrators, had overall responsibility for implementing the Adolescent Anaemia Prevention Programme. Medical staff provided services in school clinics and at HIO health care facilities.

B. Process and progress

Phase 1

In September 1999, the first phase of the project commenced in 84 schools located in the Fayoum Governorate, with the aim of reaching 70 000 students. A two-pronged approach was adopted for the programme: supplementation and dietary improvement through nutrition education, both with routine monitoring. Prior to the programme launch, consultations were held to seek consensus regarding the type of formulation to be used for supplements, the frequency of distribution, how to get the tablets to schools, and how to ensure compliance and monitor the consumption of tablets. It was agreed that WIFS would be promoted. In dialogue with experts, the planners were convinced that WIFS, being limited to one IFA tablet per week, would have minimal exposure and therefore subjects with thalassaemia minor would not experience harmful effects. No special effort was made to follow such cases in the project.

Operational research during the first phase in Fayoum Governate tested the efficacy of WIFS and the logistics of IFA supply, as well as the appropriateness of the mechanisms for distributing supplements, increasing compliance and monitoring consumption. In addition to operational research, qualitative research was also undertaken in the governorates of Aswan and Fayoum to develop an IEC strategy. The findings of this research were used to develop a school-based strategy for reducing the prevalence of anaemia in both adolescent boys and girls in grades 9-11.

Phase 2

The second phase was launched in February 2000 in Aswan Governorate to test the operational design of the programme. The demonstration project in Aswan reached 349 schools and about 150 000 students in 4000 classes. In this second phase, the programme was implemented with the help of additional hired staff to distribute supplements and impart health education. The job functions were clearly defined for tablet distributors and health educators. The tablet distributors were put in charge of ensuring an adequate weekly supply of supplements on fixed days, supervising and recording consumption and compliance data at the school level. Depending on the size of the school, one or two SHIP health visitors or nurses were assigned to schools for tablet distribution. Tablet distribution required 10-15 minutes in a class of about 45 students.

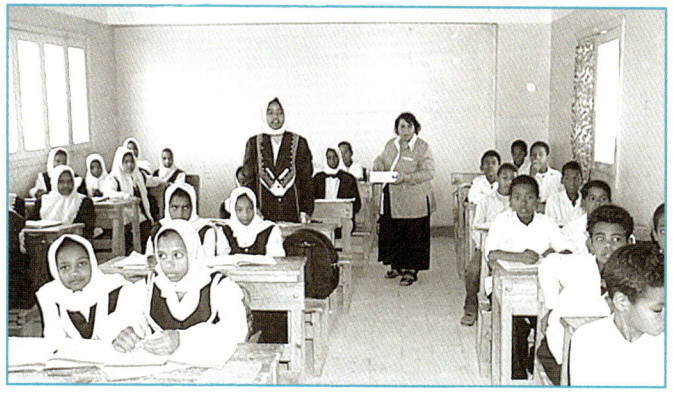

Iron tablet distribution in secondary school

Operational research was conducted with 64 students to test WIFS compliance during the month of Ramadan, when students are fasting and are unable to eat or drink during the day. This is one month of the year when the IFA supplement cannot be taken at school. Children were therefore supplied with IFA tablets and instructed to take the tablet one to two hours after they broke their fast at home. All but one of the 64 students regularly consumed the tablet. Forgetfulness was addressed by placing the tablet on the TV, table or bed pillow. The findings of research revealed that WIFS could be continued during Ramadan if appropriate education was provided.

A cadre of health educators, young university graduates, often inexperienced and with no medical background, was involved in conducting nutrition education sessions and education campaigns. These health educators were selected through a rigorous process and were trained to effectively relate to adolescents, conduct interactive sessions, answer questions about anaemia and motivate students to consume tablets. A total of 21 health educators and one supervisor were appointed for the health education task in the Aswan Governorate. Each health educator was assigned 16 schools.

Phase 3

In the third phase, in 2001, adolescent boys and girls from preparatory and secondary schools (public, private, religious, government and technical schools) from the five Upper Egypt governorates (Aswan, Beni-Suef, Fayoum, Luxor and Qena) participated in the Adolescent Anaemia Prevention Programme. The goal was to reduce existing anaemia rates and prevent anaemia in adolescent boys and girls through the well-proven two-pronged strategy. The national school enrolment was 73%, with variation by sex and locale. Evidence of the effectiveness of the demonstration project during the first two phases was used for advocacy to gain political commitment.

In the scaling-up phase, the strategy of WIFS distribution was further modified. The Ministry of Education was involved, and the responsibility for tablet distribution was handed over to teachers, since it was noted during the demonstration phase that the tasks were better performed with the assistance of teachers and other school staff. Moreover, distribution through the network of schoolteachers was also observed to increase the sustainability of the programme when taken to scale. Community participation was obtained through the involvement of district officials.

A two-pronged approach was adopted for anaemia prevention — WIFS and improvement in diet through nutrition education. Deworming was not included as an intervention in the programme since a national programme to screen and treat schistosomiasis in schoolchildren was fully operational. Political recognition and priority was considered critical. The roles of the two ministries, Health and Education, were well defined. The Health Department was essentially made responsible for supplying the supplements, while the Education Department was in charge of health and nutrition education, distribution of tablets and monitoring of consumption. The Ministry of Education agreed to implement tablet distribution under the supervision of SHIP.

For work with schools, a systematic database of schools, classes and students was compiled, with collaboration from the Ministry of Education. Those data were used for planning the intervention, with a specific focus on provision of WIFS and nutrition education for dietary improvement. Staff from the Ministry of Education and the Ministry of Health and Population held numerous district-level planning meetings to ensure that the anaemia programme was adapted to the local district situation. Community involvement was ensured with meetings with governorate and district health officials.

IFA supply

The IFA supplement formula was selected from the National Essential Drug List and contained 60 mg of elemental iron (200 mg ferrous fumarate) and 0.3 mg of folic acid. Tablets were initially yellow in colour but, during the expansion phase, the colour of the tablet was changed to red to relate to "strengthening of the blood". Tablets were purchased from an approved government pharmacy and were distributed directly from the government pharmacy to the HIO and then on to district warehouses. The district SHIP was responsible for distributing the monthly supply of IFA tablets to school clinics, as well as for providing the cups of water (75ml) required for swallowing tablets. SHIP received support from the Ministry of Health and Population for transportation of the supplies.

As per the agreed strategy, distribution and consumption of IFA supplements was undertaken on a fixed day of the week — the first day of every week, when attendance at school was noted to be highest. In cases where a student was absent on the IFA distribution day, a record was maintained and the student was followed up to ensure consumption of supplements within the same week.

IEC activities

Along with WIFS distribution, an effort was made to encourage cooperation between teachers and health workers and to increase student and public awareness of anaemia through the mass media.

Qualitative research, involving focus group discussions and trials of improved practices, was undertaken with adolescent boys and girls in both rural and urban locations to help develop a successful IEC strategy and create demand for WIFS. Separate focus group discussions were held with adolescent boys and girls, as well as mothers. Information was sought regarding the public's understanding of: good nutrition, anaemia, iron supplements and healthy diets. Furthermore, information regarding effective media channels, feasible dietary changes and methods of influencing change in dietary practices was gathered.

The formative research revealed that messages about iron would be most convincing if they focused on school performance, energy, physical growth and mental development, since Egyptian families accord very high significance to education. Regarding dietary practices, there was a special focus on the following four key messages: not skipping breakfast, consuming iron-rich food with each meal, eating fruit and vegetables rich in vitamin C, and not consuming tea for at least one hour after a meal.

A communication strategy was developed with the following key components at three critical levels:

- In-school activities (campaigns, self-instructional school booklets, posters and non-formal educational activities, weekly messages from tablet distributors).
- At-home reinforcement (instructional reminders for mothers).
- Community awareness (television spots).

The school activities were developed so that no materials or teaching aids were required and they included things such as playing games that relied on information about nutrition and anaemia to win.

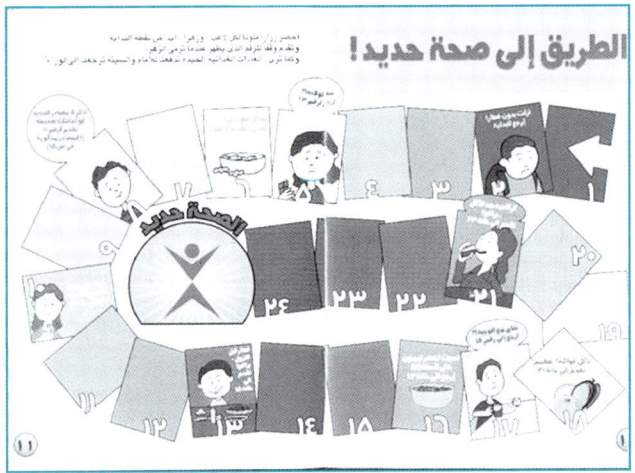

Game from the preparatory student booklet.
The aim is to achieve iron health.

A colourful poster in each classroom and a self-instructional booklet for each student supported health education sessions. The booklet contained interactive stories, word games and puzzles based on information about anaemia. *A Nutrition and health educator's guide* provided complete information on implementing the school programme for health educators. Pamphlets on anaemia and its prevention through diet and supplements were distributed to mothers.

A week prior to the launch of the programme, the headmaster of each school announced the programme's activities and the importance of WIFS for health, growth and educational achievement. Television spots on local government channels, with information on the Anaemia Programme and WIFS, were also used to promote the programme. Broadcasts also helped dispel any rumours or suspicions regarding IFA supplements being associated with birth pills or bad side-effects. Airing of the spots was started a month prior to the launch of the programme in schools and continued throughout the school year. The distribution of IFA tablets on a weekly basis also motivated consumption of WIFS and reinforced healthy dietary behavioural practices.

Monitoring

A system was developed by the project team to monitor tablet distribution and compliance. In the initial phase, the tablet distributors played a central role in monitoring consumption and compliance. The distributors were responsible for maintaining a class record and school register and forwarding the record to district staff. At the governorate level, a special computerized sheet was used for entering district data. Spreadsheets from governorates were further compiled into specific monthly monitoring reports at the central SHIP office. Care was taken to have simple recording formats and registers requiring very little effort in documentation. The system was tested in 54 schools and adjustments were made to streamline procedures.

Additionally, a periodic review of programme progress, with a view to identifying constraints that might require correction, was undertaken through a sentinel surveillance system. As per the surveillance system, a survey was undertaken before programme implementation and was repeated at the end of each school year to study iron status; anaemia prevalence; WIFS consumption; anthropometry (height and weight); and knowledge, attitudes and practices related to four key behaviours (not skipping breakfast, consumption of iron-rich food with each meal, eating fruit and vegetables rich in vitamin C and not consuming tea for at least one hour after a meal).

Training

Changes in education and training methodology were introduced, with a greater emphasis on dealing with larger groups: introducing activity-based education sessions, adjusting the curriculum and increasing the focus on developing skills in influencing behavioural change in the adolescent population. Training of health and education staff focused primarily on developing skills and communicating the minimum technical information considered critical for IEC activities and counselling. A 14-day training session was organized for health educators, conducted by a team who were prepared as master trainers by IEC experts. The educators were trained on how to deal with large groups, how to be effective trainers of adolescents, the logistics of conducting the programme and reporting requirements. Primary focus was not given to scientific aspects. Tablet distributors were trained in the technique of distribution, logistics and recording.

Evaluation

Data were collected before the implementation phase and three months post-implementation in 10 sentinel schools in Aswan. Two classes of students from each school were selected randomly. The total matched sample was 608 students. WIFS was shown to be effective among both adolescent boys and girls in reducing anaemia by 20% in a period of three months, decreasing from 30% to 24% (Figure 8). In boys, anaemia prevalence fell from 36% to 32%, and in girls from 24% to 17.5%.

Figure 8: Prevalence of anaemia among 1st level secondary students by sex; pre-supplementation and three months post-supplementation assessments

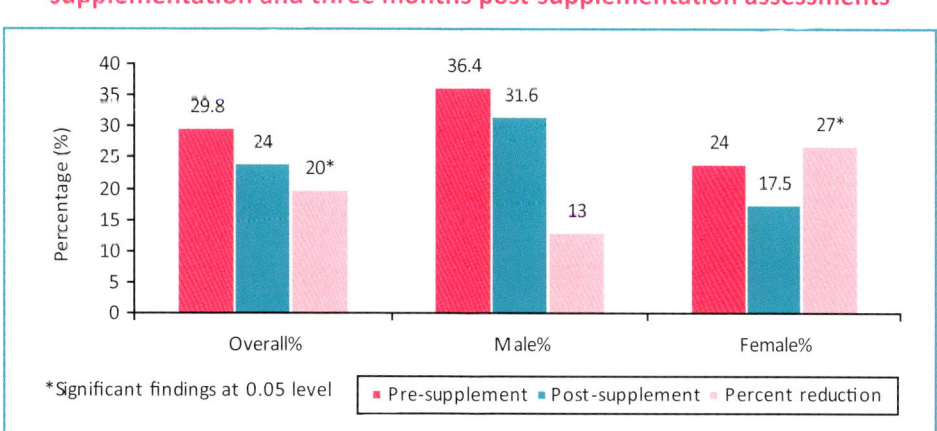

Mild anaemia was most common (Figure 9). The overall decrease in girls was significant. Moderate anaemia in girls was higher than in boys, and, with intervention, it was reduced by more than 44%. The decrease in moderate anaemia was significant. In addition, nutrition education had a significant effect on knowledge, attitudes and practices regarding the prevention of iron deficiency.

Figure 9: Prevalence of anaemia among 1st level secondary students by severity of anaemia; pre-supplementation and three months post-supplementation assessments

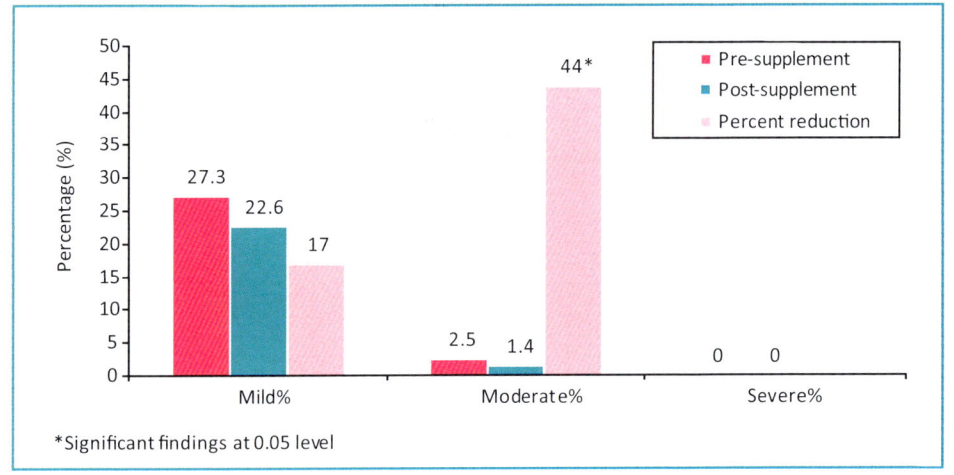

*Significant findings at 0.05 level

Compliance

Compliance was very high. In the first governorate (Aswan), only 1% of students refused to take WIFS. The refusal rate in fact dropped as implementation time increased and this was associated with the influence of nutrition education and delivery of information on prevention of anaemia. The average number of tablets received by each participating student in the first month was 2.79, while after two months it increased to 3.8 per student. It was evident that providing nutrition and health education helped overcome resistance and improved acceptance of iron supplementation.

> It was evident that providing nutrition and health education helped overcome resistance and improved acceptance of iron supplementation.

The success of the programme was attributed to gaining political support and the motivation of programme personnel. This was possible since evidence of programme efficacy was documented and used to influence politicians and policy-makers. The project proved that a two-pronged strategy comprising of WIFS and well-planned, intensive health education is effective in preventing anaemia in adolescent populations in schools. Providing nutrition and health education improves acceptance of iron supplementation. In areas, where resistance to supplementation is high, education activities should precede supplementation. Implementing non-formal educational modules in formal school settings is effective and provides the opportunity to reach a larger number of students.

Based on the successful module, the Government of Egypt launched the WIFS programme as a joint collaboration between the Ministry of Health and Population and HIO in 2003. Each organization bears 50% of the cost, the Ministry covering the cost of the IFA tablets and HIO covering the cost of training, printing of educational materials, cups for water and coordination meetings. The supplement used for the WIFS programme contains 120 mg of ferrous fumarate and 0.3 mg of folic acid, and costs US$ 026-0.31 for an annual supply of 52 tablets. The cost of implementation was reduced from US$ 0.50/child/year to US$ 0.36 /child/year in 2004-2005. Since February 2008, the Adolescent Anaemia Prevention Programme has covered 6 million schoolchildren; both girls and boys aged 10-20 years. In addition to this programme, the Ministry of Health covers 1 million WRA.

5.2 Lessons learnt

- Documenting evidence of programme efficacy is useful to influence politicians and policy-makers and gain their support. Programme success is dependent on political support and motivated programme personnel.
- To prevent anaemia, a two-pronged approach, comprising WIFS and nutrition education activities, is needed. WIFS addresses the immediate problem, while nutrition education is a long-term solution.
- Involvement of the two primary ministries, the Ministry of Health and Population and the Ministry of Education, is critical for effective implementation. Defining the division of responsibilities between the two ministries is crucial for programme success.
- Formative research, such as focus group discussions and trials of improved practices, are useful for understanding the knowledge, attitudes and practices of adolescent boys and girls and their mothers regarding anaemia, WIFS and dietary practices. Additionally, formative research could be used to identify methods for motivating students and caregivers to adopt correct preventive measures for anaemia.
- Supplying WIFS to nodal government departments, if ensured through a government pharmacy, helps to improve the sustainability of the WIFS programme. Pilot-testing of the logistic system is important prior to scaling up.
- The presentation and colour of IFA tablets for the WIFS programme should be distinct so that they are not perceived as birth control pills. Red is a more acceptable colour than yellow, since red is associated with "strengthening of the blood". Moreover, red is preferred to yellow when birth pills are yellow.
- A fixed-day strategy is effective for managing WIFS programmes. Monday was considered the most appropriate fixed day, since school attendance of students was highest on the first day of the week. Moreover, an opportunity is available to reach students within the week if they are absent on Mondays.
- The distribution process for WIFS is smoother using a network of teachers and it increases the sustainability of the programme when taken to scale. During WIFS distribution, the availability of water for swallowing should be ensured.
- During the one-month Ramadan period, WIFS can continue to be consumed at home by students if they are provided with a supply of IFA and are educated to consume IFA supplements about two hours after breaking their fast.
- Planning a communication strategy, based on formative research, is effective. Positioning the message for promoting WIFS in terms of learning and education, school performance, energy, physical growth and mental development is more acceptable and convincing to students and the community.

- It is important to raise awareness regarding prevention of anaemia and the significance of both dietary improvement and WIFS prior to launching the Anaemia Prevention Programme.

- Three levels of communication activities complement and reinforce the messages on anaemia prevention: school activities using participatory techniques (in-school campaigns, self-instructional school booklets, posters, non-formal educational activities, weekly educational sessions) along with administration of WIFS); home-level activities (instruction reminders for mothers); and community-level awareness actions (informative television spots). To sustain such educational activities, it is crucial to develop health education activities that require no materials or teaching aids e.g. playing games, creating a soap opera.

- When a programme is conducted at a national or sub-national level it is able to use TV spots on local government channels. Airing of the spots should be started a month prior to the launch of the programme in schools and continued throughout the school year.

- Young university graduates are well accepted by adolescents and can therefore be hired for local health education activities. Selection criteria and a well-defined hiring process are essential. These educators, with appropriate training, can effectively relate to adolescents, conduct interactive sessions, deal with large groups and respond to questions on anaemia.

- To maintain distribution records, class and school registers are practical. The lay-out of registers should be simple to facilitate entry of information and data. The design and content of registers must be field-tested prior to introducing it as a recording tool. It is useful to discuss progress at monthly meetings with stakeholders to identify and solve problems. Such meetings also facilitate cooperation among stakeholders.

- Software is needed for compilation of monitoring data on WIFS at governorate or district level to facilitate analysis and action.

- Through dialogue with experts, the planners in the Egypt programme were convinced that WIFS, being limited to one IFA tablet per week, would not have any harmful effects for subjects with thalassaemia minor, a common condition in several countries where malaria was or still is a public health problem. This aspect is of interest for other countries where thalassaemia is common.

References

1. Egypt's adolescent anaemia prevention programme: a report on programme development, pilot efforts and lessons learned. Cairo, Ministry of Health and Population, Health Insurance Organization, 1998.

2. Dr Nagwa El Ashry, General Director, School Age Health Care Department, Ministry of Health, Personal email communication of 2 August 2009.

5.3 Egypt WIFS Programme – A summary

Time framework and coverage	Age group	Anaemia prevalence	Intervention package	Nodal implementing agencies	Impact	Current status
• Phase launched Sept 1999 — one governate, 84 schools, 70 000 students • Phase 2 launched February 2000 — 2 governorates, 349 schools, 150 000 students • Phase 3 — 5 governorates of Upper Egypt — from 2008, 6 million students targeted	11-19 years. Both boys and girls (only programme with boys).	30% adolescents, grades 9-11	• WIFS • Nutrition education for dietary improvement. (Deworming was excluded since a national programme to screen and treat schistosomiasis was already in operation.)	• Health department • Social health insurance programme (SHIP) • Department of Maternal, Child Health, Ministry of Health and Population • Ministry of Education	• Anaemia reduced by 20% in six months in both boys and girls	• Since February 2008, the Government has launched: 1. Prevention of Anaemia in WRA by Ministry of Health and Population — covers 1 million WRA. 2. Prevention of Anaemia in Adolescence through schools (10-20 year-old girls and boys) — launched in 2003, now covers 6 million adolescents.

Supply and consumption of WIFS

Composition, packaging and supply procurement	Cost	Specific approach used	Specific consumption instructions	IFA Supply to recipients		Access	Supervision during WIFS consumption
				Free / purchased			
• IFA supplement – 60 mg of elemental iron as ferrous sulphate, 0.3 mg of folic acid. • Formulation for supplement selected from the national essential drug list. • Red colour tablets. Red colour used since associated with strengthening of blood and red tablet will not be mistaken for birth pills. • Health Department in charge of supplying the supplements. • Tablets purchased from an approved government pharmacy supplied to Health insurance Organization (HIO).	Not presented for the case study #	• Fixed day – Mondays (attendance at school highest. Easy to follow up absent students within the week.)	• Not to consume tea for at least one hour after a meal. • Along with supplements, cups (75 ml) were supplied for provision of water for swallowing.	• No cost	• Monthly supply to school	• Education department (teachers) in charge of distribution. • Teachers in charge of class distribution (distribution to 45 students takes 15 minutes.)	• By teachers and SHIP representatives.

cost of tablets in 2009 was US$ 0.28-0.31 for 52 tablets. Cost of Programme in 2002-2003 was US$ 0.50 /school child / year and, in 2004-2005, US$ 0.36 / school child /year

Efforts to increase compliance (IEC / Social mobilization / Strategy)

Positive attributes / benefits experienced	Side-effects reported and managed	Supplement-promotion strategy	Compliance
	• Nutrition and health education prior to launch of the project and throughout the project resulted in greater acceptance of iron supplementation. • Rumours dispelled regarding birth pills and side-effects.	• A qualitative research study preceded development of the communication strategy. • Young university graduates were trained as health educators initially. Later replaced by teachers. • Messages positioned to focus on health, school performance, energy, physical growth and mental development. • Focus on four key dietary behaviours: not skipping breakfast, consuming iron-rich food with each meal, eating fruits and vegetables rich in vitamin C, not consuming tea for at least one hour after meal. • Activities: raising awareness among students through school campaigns, self-instruction booklets, posters and non-formal education activities. • Instructional reminder to mothers – pamphlets for mothers. • Increased public awareness through mass media – TV spots. • Community awareness through mass media. • Implementing non-formal education module in formal school setting is effective. • IEC materials include colourful class posters, self-instruction booklets, interactive stories, games and puzzles. • Three levels of IEC: school-based, home-level reinforcement and community-level awareness. • Nutrition and health education guide used by teachers and other workers.	Compliance reported as 92.2% in phase 1. Compliance increased with time of implementation i.e. refusal to take WIFS dropped with increase in time of implementation.

Training and monitoring

Training	Monitoring Individual cards / registers etc	Other positive contributing factors
• Focus of training: training focused on: dealing with larger groups, organizing activity-based education sessions and interactive sessions, skills in influencing behavioural change in an adolescent population, and monitoring records, plus minimal technical information. Techniques for distribution, logistics and recording. Scientific aspects were not given primary focus.	• Simple class and school monitoring formats and registers for recording compliance. • District-level – a special computerized sheet for compliance and a computerised system at district, governorate and national levels. • Periodic reviews of programme progress.	• High level of political support. • Involvement of two ministries, with well defined responsibilities. • Continuous IFA supply.

6. The Lao People's Democratic Republic

6.1 WIFS demonstration project among women of child-bearing age

PROJECT AT A GLANCE	
Date of programme	• October 2006 – April 2007
Location	• Lamam district, Sekong Province
Number of participants	• 2160 schoolgirls and WRA
Project managed by	• Hygiene and Prevention Department, Ministry of Health
Reduction in anaemia rate	• 61.5% in schoolgirls over a six-month period • 38.9% in WRA over a six-month period
Compliance rate	• 74.3%
Programme costs	• US$10-12 / WRA — estimated cost in the pilot phase based on total project cost divided by number of WRA covered

A. Project design

Background

The Lao People's Democratic Republic has a population of 5.6 million, with 72.8% of the people living in rural areas. Maternal mortality and low birth weight are significant problems in the country and anaemia is recognized as a major contributing factor. As per the National Nutrition Survey, 2006, the prevalence of anaemia in the reproductive age is high, with 36.2% of all WRA anaemic and 23.2% having iron-deficiency anaemia with ferritin levels below 15mcg/l. ID is recognized to be the most common cause of nutritional anaemia. The primary cause of ID has been attributed to insufficient intake of iron-rich foods, such as meat and green leafy vegetables, and high rates of infectious diseases and intestinal parasitic infections.

The country, therefore, introduced intervention measures to address IDA. The intervention was limited to provision of a daily IFA supplement from months four to nine of pregnancy (180 days/tablets) and post delivery for three months (90 tablets of IFA). In 2000, the iron supplementation programme was studied and found to be unsatisfactory, with coverage of daily dosage reported to be as low as 13.0%. Moreover, iron supplementation following the onset of pregnancy was considered to be a late intervention, since available data indicated that many women were already anaemic or iron-deficient when their pregnancies began. In addition, early marriage and conception during adolescence were reported to be common, with many rural adolescent girls marrying at around 17 years of age. It was therefore considered important to introduce preventive measures prior to the onset of pregnancy or even earlier, during adolescence. In fact, introducing intervention measures for prevention of anaemia during adolescence was considered critical, not only to positively influence reproductive performance, but also for its impact on growth, school performance and morbidity status. An operational trial project on WIFS was therefore launched for WRA.

The demonstration programme was implemented between October 2006 and April 2007 in three phases. Phase 1 focused on collecting baseline data on

> **Iron supplementation following the onset of pregnancy was considered to be a late intervention, since available data indicated that many women were already anaemic or iron-deficient when their pregnancies began.**

haemoglobin levels and knowledge, attitudes and practices, with the help of trained programme-change agents. Phase 2 was the implementation period, including supervision and monitoring. Evaluation of programme performance was undertaken in Phase 3.

The project covered nine villages and four secondary schools in the Lamam district of Sekong Province, in the southern part of the country. The nodal implementing department was the Hygiene and Prevention Department of the Ministry of Health, supported by WHO and the Institute of Public Health. The latter was responsible for data management and analysis. The nodal department cooperated with various other departments at the provincial and district levels viz. the Provincial Department of Health, the Directorate of Secondary Schools, the Provincial Women's Union, and Mother and Child Services.

Project objectives

The general objective of the project was to determine the effect of WIFS on the anaemia status of WRA in Sekong Province after a period of seven months. The specific objectives were:

- to prove the effectiveness of WIFS in reducing anaemia among Lao WRA;
- to investigate sustainable delivery methods for WIFS for WRA using three distribution channels in rural communities: village health volunteers, the Women's Union and schoolteachers; and
- to support the introduction of WIFS in MCH policy to solve the problem of IDA and explore the feasibility of this approach in view of a possible larger-scale intervention.

Project roles and responsibilities

The programme design was developed by integrating WIFS into the ongoing WHO-supported programme on Primary Health Care in Sekong Province. The administration of WIFS was started immediately after the baseline survey. Staff of the Sekong Provincial Hospital and Lamam District were involved as the two coordinators, one for the provincial and one for the district level. Their roles primarily included managing the budget for incentives given to change agents (CAs), monitoring visits to villages once a month, and facilitating implementation. During visits to the villages, the Provincial Coordinators supported CAs in conducting nutrition education sessions, collected information and discussed problems regarding WIFS supply, distribution, consumption and compliance. Reports on these field visits were produced on a monthly basis and shared with the main coordinator at the central level.

CAs included teachers in schools, village Women's Union leaders and village health volunteers. All CAs, both male and female, were given a six-month supply of IFA supplements, which they distributed to WRA in the community as well as in schools on the fixed supplement day. Two teachers per school functioned as CAs, while nine members of the Women's Union and nine village health volunteers contacted women in the communities of nine selected project villages. It was estimated that one village health volunteer would be able to distribute supplements to about 52 WRA, while one teacher would distribute IFA supplements to 150 schoolchildren.

It was estimated that one village health volunteer would be able to distribute supplements to about 52 WRA, while one teacher would distribute IFA supplements to 150 schoolchildren.

Mobilization of local leaders was recognized as being important for successful implementation. A special effort was therefore made to seek their support and ensure communication among programme leaders. To obtain the support of community leaders, field visits to villages where the programme was being implemented were organized for village leaders and the chief of the Women's Union. To launch the school programme, a special event was organized in one of the four project schools.

B. Process and progress

IFA supply

Supplies of WIFS were procured, in accordance with the formula recommended by WHO. The supply was produced and donated by United Laboratories (UNILAB), Manila, the Philippines. The WIFS tablets were referred to as "Femina" and contained 60 mg of elemental iron and 3.5 mg of folic acid. A fixed-day approach was used for WIFS distribution and consumption — every Monday of the week was fixed for iron supplementation. Women in the age group 12-49 years (WRA) were advised to take the supplement with clean drinking water.

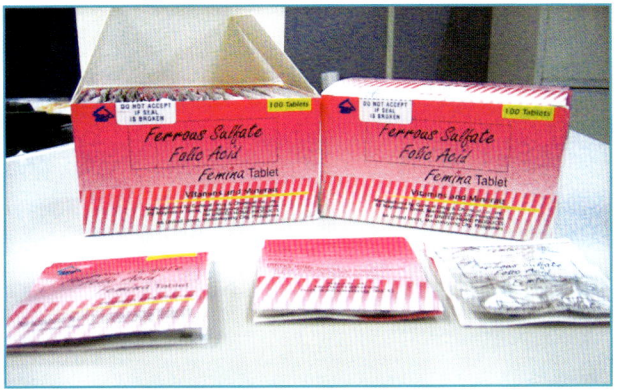

Product shot of Femina tablets

The tablets were taken immediately after receiving the supplement from the CAs and, as far as possible, in the presence of the CAs. In cases where women were not available on Mondays due to fieldwork, distribution and consumption was organized on other days especially for them. Each woman was also given 500 mg of mebendazole prior to starting WIFS since the prevalence of intestinal parasite infection in the area was known to be very high, with 62% of primary-school children suffering from worm infestation.

IEC activities

The IEC strategy positioned the supplement, not just as a medicine to prevent and cure anaemia, but also as a positive intervention for improving the quality of life. The emphasis was on shifting the focus to the fact that:

> *'All women experience physical, mental and emotional changes as they go through life stages, especially during their reproductive years (from menarche to menopause). All women in this stage of the life cycle should take WIFS together with improved diets, to enhance their well-being and prevent IFA deficiency.'*

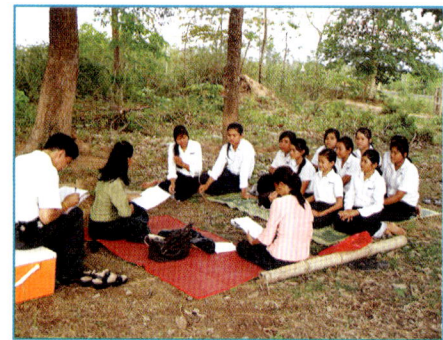
Schoolgirls participating in the WIFS Programme

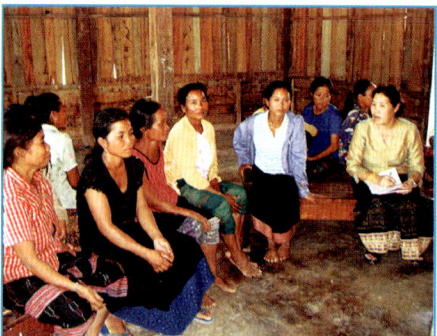
Training of change agents (CAs)

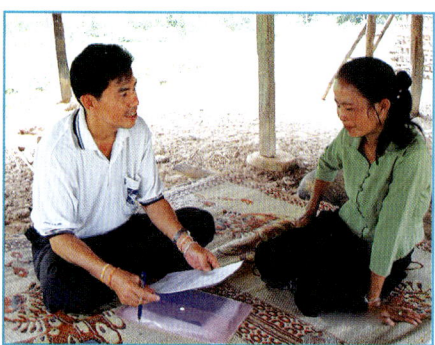
Male change agent counselling a WRA

Training

Training was organized for all CAs, including teachers, by a team of officers from the Ministry of Health. The contents of the two-day training included information on:

- the problem of anaemia in the country;
- the link between iron status and low birth weight;
- measures to prevent iron deficiency;
- iron-rich food sources;
- the significance of WIFS;
- the application of experiences and lessons learnt from WIFS programmes in other countries;
- actions to address side-effects following WIFS administration;
- the importance of deworming;
- the critical role of community involvement for the success of the project;
- the role of change agents; and
- the use of monthly and six-monthly monitoring formats.

All CAs were provided with printed information and educational materials during training and were shown how to use them effectively during health education sessions. Interestingly, a few selected CAs, primarily teachers, were also involved in the initial stage of development and production of IEC materials through small informal workshops held by programme coordinators.

Monitoring and compliance

CAs developed a standard format for recording information on compliance on a weekly basis. At the end of each month, coordinators from the provincial and district levels visited the villages and schools. A dialogue was maintained between the project team and community leaders and this was found to be extremely useful in sustaining interest in the project. During these monthly monitoring visits, health education sessions were also conducted and the opportunity was taken to address the issue of side-effects.

A total of 26 CAs, comprising teachers, village Women's Union members and village health volunteers, were involved in focus group discussions. The CAs were given a small monetary incentive of US$8/person/month and other benefits in the form of refresher training, provision of stationary and educational materials, as well as the opportunity to visit other projects for study purposes.

The CAs, including teachers and their spouses, were also encouraged to consume WIFS, to convince them further of the benefits of IFA supplements. This strategy was effective, not only in demonstrating the importance of regular consumption of WIFS and promoting its consumption, but also in gaining the confidence of the community.

The CAs distributed the supplements free of charge and regularly interacted with the community. No special advice was given regarding the preferred time for taking the tablets. School students normally consumed WIFS at around 4:30 in the afternoon every Monday, before finishing class or before going home, while village women, depending on what was more suitable, took the tablet in the morning before or after lunch. The CAs discussed side-effects with adolescents and women. The village women were encouraged to make their own arrangements for consumption of tablets since it was noted that administration of WIFS by CAs to a group of women would result in logistical problems, such as arranging a supply of clean water for swallowing the tablets. Group administration of WIFS to village women was therefore not viewed as a practical strategy, despite recognition that consumption could be better supervised.

In a period of six months, 930 WRAs and 1230 schoolgirls were covered. Monthly monitoring visits and data-recording by provincial coordinators were given special attention to increase compliance and effective follow-up.

Evaluation

The impact of seven months of WIFS implementation was assessed by the Hygiene and Prevention Department of the Ministry of Health. It was noted that education sessions had a significant impact on the knowledge of adolescent girls and women regarding causes of anaemia and preventive measures (Figure 10).

Figure 10: Change in women's knowledge on the causes of anaemia following the intervention

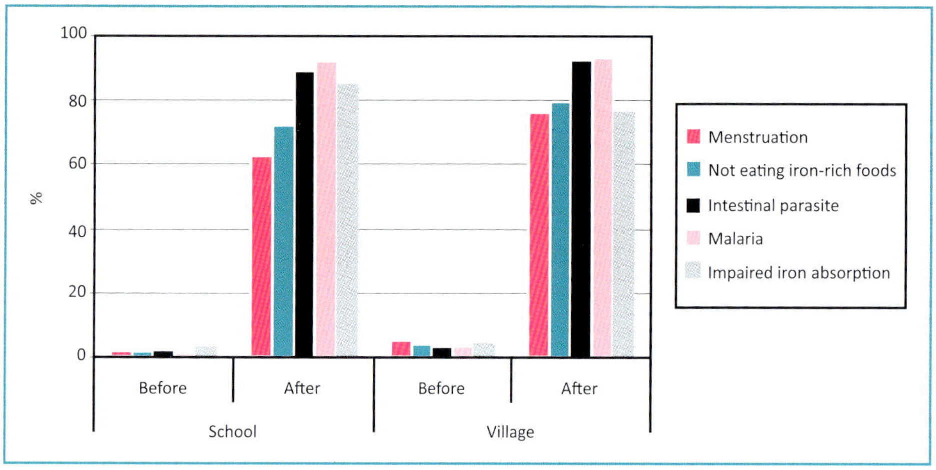

Over a period of seven months, over 90% of the target population had received supplements and this was attributed, to a great extent, to the active participation of the CAs. An exploratory exercise was undertaken to estimate the price women would be prepared to pay for the supplements. This revealed that 67.9% would be ready to pay US$ 0.05 per tablet. However, taking into consideration the fact that the majority of the population is poor, tablets continued to be distributed free of charge.

Women and students reported positive benefits after taking the supplements. The students who participated in the project reported that the regular use of WIFS resulted in them feeling stronger, having better sleep, increased energy, increased appetite, improved concentration and an increased capacity to work and earn. Village women also reported benefits, such as reduced illness and therefore financial benefits, improved appetite and weight gain, increased energy to work, and regularization of their menstruation cycles, as well as improved skin appearance. Students and women often communicated these benefits to others in the community.

The impact of WIFS on anaemia status was studied by the Hygiene and Prevention Department and the Institute of Public Health. A baseline survey was undertaken of 936 randomly selected women and a follow-up study of 615 of these women was conducted after a period of six months. The decrease in the number of WRA surveyed the second time was due to such reasons as transfer of residency, women being unavailable because they were too busy in the fields or with household chores, fear of blood tests, and students not being at school. Haemoglobin was measured using the HemoCue method. Anaemia in women was defined as Hb below 120 g/L. In a period of six months, the overall prevalence of anaemia in schools and villages was found to have decreased from 43% to 23%. In schools, 33.8% of girls were anaemic prior to the intervention and this had decreased to 13%, while in the community the 48.6% of women who were anaemic at baseline had fallen to 29.7%.

In a period of six months, the overall prevalence of anaemia in schools and villages decreased from 43% to 23%.

Figure 11: Anaemia prevalence in schools and villages before and after intervention

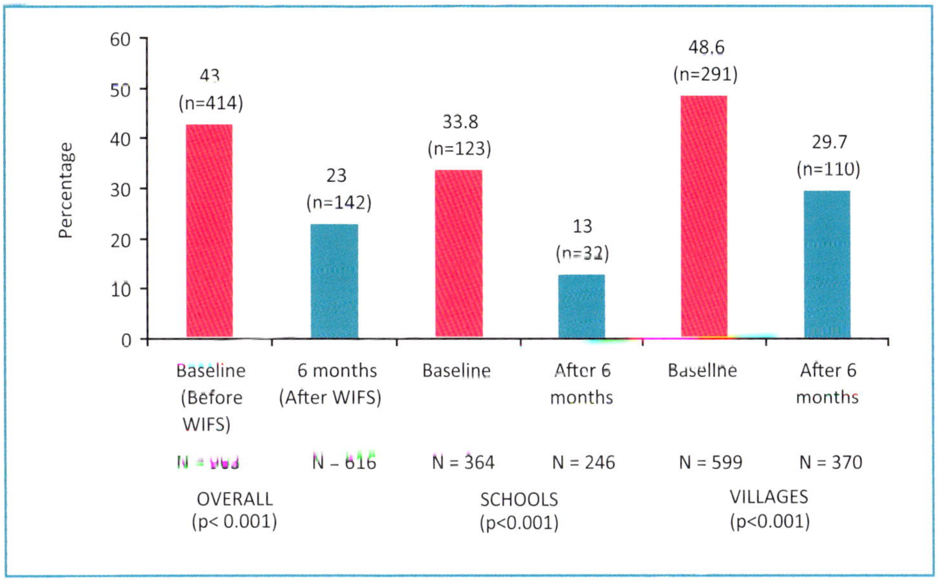

	OVERALL (p< 0.001)	SCHOOLS (p<0.001)	VILLAGES (p<0.001)
Baseline	43 (n=414), N=963	33.8 (n=123), N=364	48.6 (n=291), N=599
After 6 months	23 (n=142), N=616	13 (n=32), N=246	29.7 (n=110), N=370

The impact of WIFS on anaemia prevalence was significant in both schools and villages. However, the reduction was much better in schools (61.5%) then in villages (38.9%). This could be attributed to the fact that the consumption of supplements was more regular in schools. Moreover, nutrition education sessions were better organized, resulting in high compliance. It was also noted that the side-effects reported at baseline had decreased by almost 50% in the endline survey. A total of 74.5% of WRA were found to have taken the recommended number of tablets, with consumption comparatively poor in older age groups, farmers and non-school women. The causes of poor compliance were primarily forgetfulness (50%), onset of pregnancy (16.7%), and side-effects such as stomach-ache (4.5%) and vomiting (1.3%). Other reasons mentioned for not taking the supplements included: working on farms, loss of appetite and fear of weight gain.

During the seven-month post-implementation review, the system for distributing supplements, as well as constraints in implementing the WIFS strategy, were reviewed. The CAs indicated that, since the majority of village people are poor and have no capacity to pay, free distribution of weekly supplements should be continued. Planned and regular use of IEC materials during nutrition education was found to be very effective. It was observed that, along with health education, monitoring and technical support should be strengthened, and actions should be taken for strong advocacy regarding the importance of WIFS.

> **Focus group discussions and the survey revealed that students considered teachers to be the best people to distribute supplements and provide counselling on the use of WIFS.**

Focus group discussions and the survey revealed that students considered teachers to be the best people to distribute supplements and provide counselling on the use of WIFS. Leaders of the village Women's Union were also considered a good choice for provision of supplements since there is one Women's Union member for every 5-10 houses and these women have the time, as well as the skills to counsel and act as CAs. However, it was observed that these CAs (influential community leaders and local promoters and implementers) of the WIFS programme should be given small monetary benefits. It was interesting to note that only some programme participants preferred the village health volunteers, since they considered them to be overloaded with other work and not always in a position to undertake the task of timely distribution. It was felt that if students and women were themselves convinced of the benefits of WIFS, they would form a critical group who would effectively convince others to take supplements and iron-rich food.

Based on the success of the pilot project, integration of the WIFS project with existing delivery systems in health, education and the private sector (factories, markets, local shops), as well as through community organizations, was proposed. It was recommended that WIFS should be provided to WRA before pregnancy, ideally beginning at menarche, especially in situations where iron-rich food sources are limited. Active efforts to involve community leaders were considered critical to the success and sustainability of the WIFS programme. Following implementation of the WIFS demonstration project, in 2009, the WIFS project model was incorporated into the National Nutrition Strategy and the National Plan of Action, as well as the essential package for Maternal and Child Care, to reduce anaemia in WRA and in pregnancy and to help reduce low birth weight and anaemia in infants.

6.2 Lessons learnt

- Of the three channels used, teachers and heads of the Women's Union are more effective for reaching WRA and promoting WIFS than village volunteers, who are often overloaded with work.
- A fixed-day approach (every Monday) plays a very important facilitating role in supply, distribution, demand creation, monitoring of consumption, follow up and compliance of WIFS.
- IEC strategies should not position WIFS as a medicine, but as a positive intervention, along with dietary improvement, to enhance the well-being of WRA and improve quality of life by preventing iron deficiency.
- Use of both male and female CAs is effective. Monetary and other incentives for CAs appear critical.
- Availability of IFA supplements should be complemented by strong health and nutrition education. Additionally, efforts must be made to ensure WIFS are made available at the very nominal price of US$US 0.05 /tablet for WRA in the community.
- Mobilization of local leaders is important for successful implementation. Organizing field visits to project sites is noted to be useful in generating interest and the leaders' support for the WIFS programme.
- Maintaining an ongoing dialogue with project teams and community leaders is helpful in sustaining interest in the project.
- Encouraging consumption of WIFS through CAs, including teachers and their spouses, results in generation of significant confidence in WRA regarding the WIFS programme and in the acceptance of WIFS as a strategy to prevent anaemia.
- Administering WIFS to women in a group is not a practical strategy, since the difficulty of logistic arrangements for providing water for swallowing tablets can outweigh the benefits of group administration, even if it provides the opportunity for supervision.

- Women often share the benefits of WIFS they have experienced with others. The advantage of building an IEC strategy linked to the benefits of WIFS is evident.
- Special attention should be given to overcoming forgetfulness, as it is the primary cause of poor compliance, especially in the community.
- Free distribution of IFA supplements is preferred by WRA, as the majority of women are poor. However, focus group studies revealed that two-thirds of women would be willing to pay between US$ 0.02 and US$0.05 per WIFS tablet.
- Planned and regular use of IEC materials is extremely important for sustaining interest in WIFS and overcoming the problem of forgetfulness, which adversely affects compliance.
- Use of a simple, standardized monitoring format is useful for regular recording of information by teachers and women leaders. Regularly entering information in the monitoring format by CAs also acts as a reminder to WRA and therefore positively influences compliance.
- Training of non-health CAs by health staff is useful in equipping them with knowledge on technical issues related to anaemia, the importance of WIFS, and sharing success stories on the impact of WIFS, as well as providing skills in communication and use of IEC materials. A training period of two days is insufficient. The use of printed training and educational materials facilitates standardization of training content.

References

1. Smitasiri S. Report of a mission to the Lao People's Democratic Republic, 15-21 October 2006. Manila, WHO Regional Office for the Western Pacific, 2006.

2. Report on evaluation of weekly iron folic acid supplementation in Sekong Province, 6 to 18 May 2007.

3. Preliminary report of operational trial of weekly iron folic acid supplementation, Sekong province, Lao People's Democratic Republic. Ministry of Health and WHO, August 2007.

4. Phengdy D, Acting Director, Mother and Child Division, Ministry of Health, Lao People's Democratic Republic, and project Team Leader: personal communications, August 2008 and July 2009.

6.3 The Lao People's Democratic Republic WIFS Programme – A summary

Time framework and coverage	Age group	Anaemia prevalence	Intervention package	Nodal implementing agencies	Impact	Current status
• Three phases • October 2006 – April 2007 Seven months of implementation in one district — nine villages and four secondary schools — 930 WRAs and 1230 schoolgirls • Scaled up to three districts with UNICEF support	12-49 years (WRA), including girls in school	In girls = 33.8% In WRA = 48.6% Overall = 43.0%	• WIFS education for dietary improvement • Mebendazole (500 mg) prior to starting WIFS	• Hygiene and Prevention Department, Ministry of Health and district departments of health, secondary schools, Women's Union.	• In a six-month period, anaemia in schoolgirls decreased by 61.5% and in WRAS by 38.9% • Overall decrease in prevalence was 53.4% — from 43% to 23%.	Following implementation of the WIFS demonstration project, in 2009 the WIFS project model was incorporated into the National Nutrition Strategy and the National Plan of Action, as well as the essential package for Maternal and Child Care, to reduce anaemia in WRA and in pregnancy and to help reduce low birth weight and anaemia in infants.

Supply and consumption of WIFS

Composition, packaging and supply procurement	Cost	Specific approach used	Specific consumption instructions	IFA Supply to recipients		Supervision during WIFS consumption
				Free / purchased	Access	
• Supply was produced and donated by UNILAB, Manila. • Each IFA tablet contained 60 mg of elemental iron + 3.5 mg of folic acid.	US$10-12 / WRA / year. Includes cost of incentives to CAs (US$8 / CA / month and estimated cost of US$2 / woman / year and US $ 0.47 / schoolgirl / year), all operational and consultancy costs. Excludes cost of IFA tablets.	• Fixed WIFS day — Monday. • If women are away in the field, an alternative date is used for WIFS. • In schools— WIFS taken in the afternoon (about 4:30 pm) before going home. • WRA — as convenient, morning or post lunch.	• Use clean water for swallowing IFA supplements.	• Distributed free of charge. • 68% women were ready to pay only US $ 0.05 / tablet.	• CAs (teachers, village Women's Union leaders, village health volunteers) received incentives. • One CA in charge of distribution to 52 WRAs and one teacher for 150 schoolchildren. • Teachers and heads of village Women's Union most acceptable and therefore considered best persons to distribute WIFS.	Supervision "as far as possible". Report indicated a wide variation in time of consumption, resulting in poor supervision. Moreover, supervision was not possible since group consumption was discouraged due to logistical problems in arranging water.

Efforts to increase compliance (IEC / Social mobilization / Strategy)

Positive attributes / benefits experienced	Side-effects reported and managed	Supplement-promotion strategy	Compliance
Positive benefits of WIFS reported by women and schoolgirls: Feeling stronger, better sleep, increase in energy, not tiring easily, increase in appetite, improvement in concentration, increase in capacity to work, regularization of menstrual cycle, improved appearance of skin and reduced illness and therefore economic impact.	Side-effects, if any, were addressed during the education sessions. Side-effects reported at baseline decreased by almost 50% after WIFS supplementation for six months.	• WIFS tablet positioned as "Femina". IEC strategy was built on benefits of WIFS. • IFA positioned, not as a medicine, but as an intervention to improve quality of life. • Women and students communicating benefits of WIFS to community. • Mobilization of local leaders – organization of field visits. Sharing of benefits experienced following consumption of WIFS. • IEC material (printed) used regularly. • CAs, including teachers, also received and consumed WIFS – resulted in gaining the confidence of the community.	• Compliance 74.5% • Contributing cause of poor compliance – forgetfulness (50%), onset of pregnancy (16.7%), side-effects: stomach ache (4.5%) and vomiting (1.3%) and others (loss of appetite, afraid of weight gain). • Monthly monitoring visits and data recording – special attention to increase compliance. • Better organized education sessions in schools – better compliance. • Regular sharing of benefits

Training and monitoring

Training	Monitoring Individual cards / registers etc	Other positive contributing factors
Training organized by the Ministry of Health for CAs (teachers, health volunteers and women leaders). The two-day training included information on anaemia, iron deficiency, dietary measures and WIFS for prevention, action to address side-effects, the significance of deworming, the critical role of CAs and lessons learnt from other WIFS project, the monitoring system and use of standard formats, the importance of community involvement, and skills in using printed information and educational materials	• Standard format for recording weekly compliance was maintained by CAs. • Monthly visit by coordinators from provincial and district levels.	• Dialogue was sustained between implementers and community leaders. • CAs were also encouraged to take WIFS to gain the confidence of the community. • The integration of the WIFS project with the existing delivery systems for health and education, as well as community organizations and private sector channels (factories, markets, local shops), was considered effective.

7. Viet Nam (Yen Bai Province)

7.1 Addressing anaemia in women through free supply of weekly iron-folic acid supplements (WIFS) and biannual administration of anti-helminth medication

	PROJECT AT A GLANCE
Date of programme	• Phase 1 – May 2006 • Phase 2 – March 2008
Location	• Yen Bai Province
Number of participants	• Estimated 250 000 WRA, 16-45 years
Project managed by	• Ministry of Health and Vietnam Institute of Malariology, Parasitology and Entomology
Reduction in anaemia rate	• 48% in a one-year period
Compliance rate	• 69% - 70%
Programme costs	• US$0.40/woman/year

A. Project design

Background

Yen Bai Province, one of the 64 provinces and cities in Viet Nam, was selected for a demonstration project addressing the public health problem of anaemia, since various surveys suggested that a high prevalence of hookworm may be one of the major causes of anaemia in the area. The province covers a mountainous region with a largely rural economy, widespread poverty and diverse ethnic groups.

The implementation plan for addressing anaemia was developed following a cross-sectional survey of a community-based sample of women living in this rural province to assess the prevalence of iron deficiency and anaemia, as well as associated risk factors. The study, undertaken in November 2005, revealed 37.5% of non-pregnant women were anaemic (Hb<120 g/L) and 23.0% were iron-deficient (Ferritin<15ng/L). Iron deficiency was more common among anaemic women, although less than one half of anaemia could be attributed to iron deficiency. Hookworm infection was present in 78.15% of women, while heavy infection was recorded in 6.3%[10]. Hookworm infection, although not found to be associated with anaemia in the population, was confirmed to be correlated with iron deficiency. The study emphasized that IDA is a major public health problem in WRA in north-west Viet Nam. Both lack of dietary iron and hookworm infection contribute to iron deficiency.

> The study emphasized that IDA is a major public health problem in WRA in north-west Viet Nam. Both lack of dietary iron and hookworm infection contribute to iron deficiency.

Target group

A one-year demonstration programme of iron supplementation and deworming was launched in May, 2006, in two districts of Yen Bai Province, Yen Binh and Tran

---

10 Casey GJ, *et al*. A free weekly iron-folic acid supplementation and regular deworming programme is associated with improved haemoglobin and iron status indicators in Vietnamese women. *BMC public health*, 2009,9(1) :261.

Yen. The programme covered 50 000 women in the reproductive age group of 16-45 years.

Programme roles and responsibilities

The 12-month intervention package consisted of WIFS and deworming. The National Institute of Malariology, Parasitology and Entomology (NIMPE) was the nodal health sector partner responsible for the project. The Department of Medicine of the University of Melbourne, Australia, and the Walter and Eliza Hall Institute of Medical Research, Australia, were the international partners. Technical support was provided by the provincial implementing agency, Yen Bai Malaria Control Programme (YBMCP), and WHO, while UNICEF supplied IFA supplements and albendazole tablets in the initial phase of the project. Financial support was also provided by a private international group, the Atlantic Philanthropies Inc. NIMPE was responsible for overseeing the implementation of the project, while YBMCP acted as the local management team[11].

An implementation plan was developed with the provincial counterparts and was approved by the Ministry of Health. Presentations of the plan were made to the Provincial People's Committee and Health Department heads to explain the purpose and value of the intervention and to ensure the active support of various authorities. Advocacy meetings were held with district heads of the Centre of Preventive Medicine and heads of commune health stations (CHS). Training sessions were organized for all village health workers (VHW) to involve them in educating women about the value of regular iron supplementation and deworming. The training was also used to involve them in implementation activities, including timely identification of constraints and resolving issues. Adoption of positive promotional practices was encouraged. The training and support of VHW was deemed essential as all the local partners identified VHW as the critical interface with WRA for successful implementation. Advocacy was facilitated by developing training and promotional materials, as well as developing a cadre of trainers. Promotional materials included posters (four copies for each village and CHS), banners for CHS and a pictorial handout with a timetable for all WRA. Advocacy efforts were intensified through the use of television media. Provincial television coverage was organized, including interviews with major partners.

Monitoring

The nodal agency for monitoring supply was the provincial implementing agency, YBMCP. Monitoring forms with information on IFA supply were received every month from CHS by YBMCP. The IFA supply was provided by YBMCP only on receipt of the completed forms with information on the stock situation. It was therefore compulsory for provincial health authorities to review information on stock and supply the status of WIFS and the deworming drug every month. Based on this information, YBMCP received a biannual supply from NIMPE.

---

11 Mihrshahi S, et al. The effectiveness of 4 monthly albendazole treatment in the reduction of soil transmitted helminth infections in women of reproductive age in Vietnam. *International journal of parasitology*, 2009, 39 (9) 1037-43.

Monitoring was undertaken routinely through regular visits to Yen Bai, including the district Preventive Medicine Centres, commune health stations and village health workers. Over the period of the project, monitoring by the core health team also contributed significantly to developing rapport among implementers at all levels. Feedback was provided by regularly submitting reports to YBMCP, who then reported to the Provincial Health Department and Provincial People's Committee. In addition, compliance was monitored by the NGO, the Research and Training Centre for Community Development (RTCCD).

B. Process and progress

IFA supply

NIMPE was responsible for ensuring a timely supply of IFA supplements and deworming tablets. IFA tablets, containing 60 mg of elemental iron as ferrous sulphate and 0.4 mg of folic acid, were initially supplied, for a year, by UNICEF. A month's supply of four brown-red, non-coated IFA tablets were packaged by the VHW in double-lidded, tamper-proof bottles for WRA.

In March 2008, the project was scaled up to the provincial level. In the scaling-up phase, the IFA supply was produced by Viet Nam-based manufacturers (NAPHACO). They were provided free of cost and were blister-packed. Albendazole (400 mg), non-coated white tablets, were supplied by UNICEF in tins of 100 tablets to each CHS, and UNICEF continued to supply them in the scaling-up phase.

The supply requirement was assessed based on target population estimates. Decentralized estimates at village level were derived from the VHW lists and forwarded to the project team. The supply channel was well defined. The tablets were procured in bulk and stored centrally at the YBMCP office. The stock was forwarded to district preventive medicine centres, who handed over the supply to CHS during monthly meetings. Flexibility in the distribution system, beyond the existing health system infrastructure, was introduced to reach WRA in remote communities where there was a lack of transport or inaccessibility due to floods, landslides or heavy rains.

CHS were responsible for handing over the IFA supply to VHW during their regular visits. Similarly, VHW informed community members and WRA when and where to access the monthly supply of WIFS, and communicated details regarding the time and venue for the supervised administration of deworming tablets. Within the village, the location and timing were standardized for distribution of the monthly supply of IFA tablets, which were free of cost. Women were counselled by VHW on the proven benefits of the intervention and were encouraged to consume the IFA tablets every week on a fixed day. Any side-effects or concerns expressed by WRA were addressed by the VHW network and communicated to the CHS. If a woman became pregnant, she was referred by a VHW to an antenatal clinic and was advised to consume daily iron supplements of a higher dose (120mg of elemental iron), supplied through the government programme.

Compliance and IEC strategies

Administration of WIFS to WRA aimed at universal coverage of all women aged 16-45 years. The consumption of WIFS was not supervised, but, to ensure high

> Community involvement was considered essential. Village health workers, being an integral part of the village community, were able to disseminate information on the positive attributes of the intervention package during social interactions.

compliance of IFA tablets, women were encouraged, by VHW, to take WIFS regularly on a designated day of the week between meals. The WRA were instructed to swallow the tablets with water and not to take the tablets on an empty stomach. WRA were also advised to avoid tea and coffee when taking the tablets. The albendazole deworming tablets on the other hand, were administered as observed treatment on locally designated days, either at CHS or in villages under the supervision of commune health workers. Women were observed for 30 minutes at each health station after administration of albendazole.

Community involvement was considered essential. VHW, being an integral part of the village community, were able to disseminate information on the positive attributes of the intervention package during social interactions. VHW were very well accepted by the community, which facilitated in generating a high level of enthusiasm among WRA. Although the project team did not select a particular day for WRA to take WIFS, VHW routinely counselled women to follow a fixed-day approach for consumption of IFA tablets. Women were warned to keep tablets away from children and this instruction was reinforced through the printed handouts distributed to WRA. In addition, to ensure a high level of community participation, the project team conducted formal and informal meetings with Women's Union leaders, commune Communist Party heads and village leaders. Occasional meetings were also organized with the Provincial People's Committee and heads of health departments to ensure the continued support and encouragement of district staff. The project team made regular trips to district centres and CHS and also held regular dialogues with VHW in order to identify problems and provide specialized support.

To encourage WIFS compliance, a handout for WRA carried the message "healthy women for healthy families" and included illustrations highlighting the significance of taking deworming medication and IFA supplements regularly for all women aged 16-45. The illustrations focused on regular deworming and iron supplements providing a healthy and happy environment for women and children. The handout carried messages about the importance of visits to CHS if a woman is pregnant or sick. The handouts also included messages cautioning users to keep the IFA tablets away from children. Posters for VHW and CHS had similar illustrations and focused on the same messages as the handout.

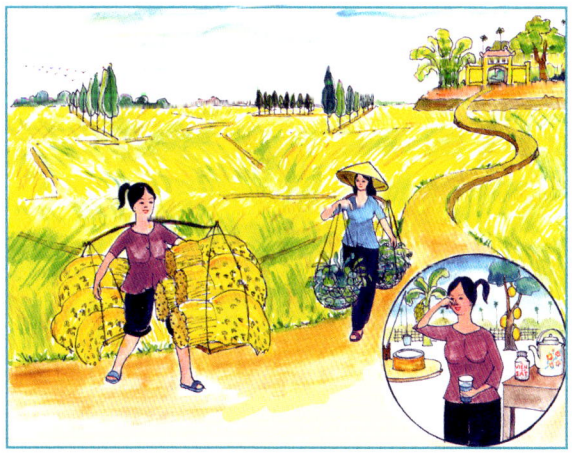

Poster with information on iron deficiency anaemia and deworming

It was considered critical to modify the IEC strategy for influencing behavioural change following the first compliance survey, conducted three months after the commencement of the intervention (August 2006) by the independent Vietnamese NGO, RTCCD. It was evident from the findings that a stronger promotional strategy was required in mountainous communes with high numbers of ethnic minority groups, who, in some cases, were suspicious of the intervention. Colourful promotional materials, including wall posters, were developed, field-tested and introduced. An informational wall calendar for WRA was also produced. The message of the calendar was that health is enhanced by taking WIFS, having a nutritious diet and wearing shoes when working in the garden. In addition, a new set of educational materials was provided to VHW to facilitate dialogue at community meetings. The additional set of posters included information on deworming, anaemia and iron deficiency. This set of posters had more detailed information on sanitary and dietary issues, causes and transmission of soil-transmitted helminth infection, and prevention and treatment of anaemia and iron deficiency. Radio programmes were produced in conjunction with the Provincial Health Communication Unit and the Voice of Viet Nam radio station. They were designed for local radio and airing over commune and village loudspeaker systems. When the programme was later expanded provincewide, the radio programmes were produced in both Vietnamese and H'mong (the predominant language in two remote districts). The television and video clips were developed by YBMCP and were screened twice weekly on provincial television. All materials were field-tested and amended prior to production and dissemination.

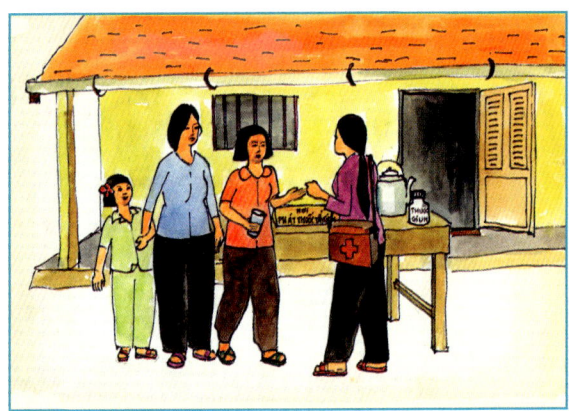

Wall poster, a promotional material targeted at WRA

In addition to intensifying promotional activities, the packaging of tablets was changed from a bottle to blister packs to increase acceptability and shelf life and to facilitate transportation. This was important since the bulk distribution of IFA tablets in double-capped bottles was neither universally approved nor found to be safe in maintaining quality. These modifications in packaging and communication strategy resulted in continued high compliance.

Training

Training and capacity-building at every level was an integral part of the project. The implementation team was trained before the intervention. The nodal health team, comprising 680 VHW from two project districts, two nurses from each CHS and two staff of each district preventive medicine centre, were trained about the causes, treatment, prevention and health risks of anaemia and hookworm infection. Training also focused on skills in administration and distribution of WIFS and albendazole, monitoring of side-effects, and follow-up with WRA. Additionally, district and commune health staff were trained in the management of IFA distribution and monitoring, as well as in maintaining a feedback mechanism regarding reported side-effects. District and commune teams were also trained in the recognition and treatment of adverse effects related to albendazole treatment. Training of senior district officers included strengthening skills in the organization of regular monthly meetings to discuss progress in project implementation with the provincial health authorities. Two training manuals in the local Vietnamese language were developed — one for trainers and the other for health staff.

Evaluation

Compliance was assessed in the two project districts using structured questionnaires in one-to-one interviews by trained interviewers. Compliance was ascertained by asking how many tablets the respondent had taken over the previous two months. The response was categorized as complete, partial or non-compliant, based on whether the consumption of WIFS was followed fully each and every week, or some but not all WIFS were consumed, or no tablets were taken. Figure 12 shows that, at three months post-intervention, in August 2006, 93% of women reported total (70%) or partial (23%) compliance with WIFS. The second monitoring survey, in September 2007, after a period of 16 months, reported that total compliance had remained consistent, with 69% reporting full compliance, while there had been a decrease in partial compliance (from 23% to 16%) and a corresponding increase in non-compliance (from 7% to 15%).

Figure 12: Compliance of WIFS by WRAs in two districts (Tran Yen and Yen Binh) of Yen Bai Province

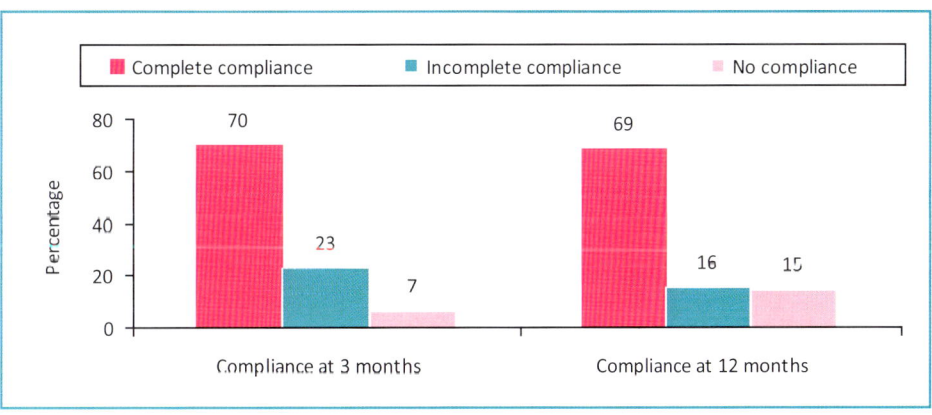

Impact evaluation revealed a significant decrease in anaemia prevalence (Hb <120 g/L) — a reduction of 48% in a period of 12 months (Figure 13). With the administration of albendazole, hookworm infection fell from 76.2% at baseline to 25.2% after 12 months of project implementation.

Figure 13: Anaemia prevalence and hookwom infestation in WRAs in two districts (Tran Yen and Yen Binh) of Yen Bai Province

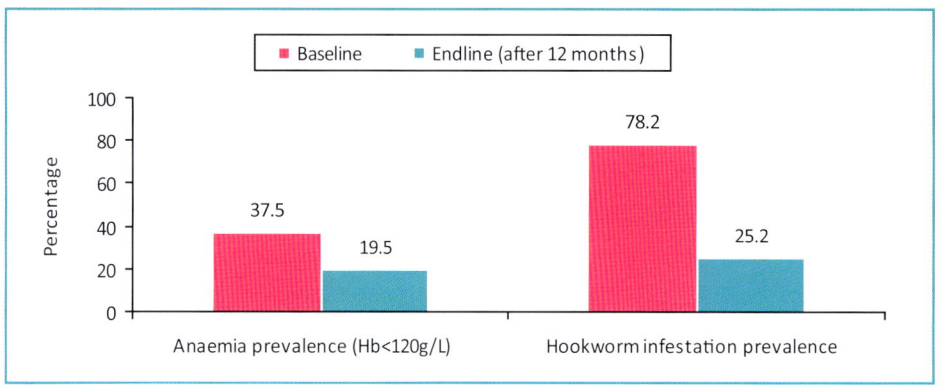

Scaling up

Based on the success of the demonstration project and its low cost, the decision was made by provincial authorities to scale up the programme to all districts of Yen Bai. In March 2008, the project was expanded across the province, to reach approximately 250 000 WRA. Commencing in August 2007, the IFA supplement was sourced as a blister pack from a Vietnamese pharmaceutical manufacturer. The blister packs were designed as six tear-off strips of five tablets per strip. Women were provided with one tear-off strip per month. Albendazole was still provided by WHO throughout the scaling-up phase, and is now given to women on a six-monthly basis. All supplements are still provided free of charge to WRA. The ownership of the project and the training of VHW have now been transferred to the provincial authorities. Community and health services continue to effectively implement the intervention. The approximate price for WIFS and biannual deworming was estimated to be only $US0.20/woman/year, using a UNICEF bulk supply at 2006 pricing. New estimates based on locally manufactured, blister-pack IFA tablets at 2008 pricing, puts the cost at $US0.40/woman/ year.

With the low cost of implementation and the positive impact on women's health, presentations to the Government of Viet Nam, via the Ministry of Health, for support and expanded distribution are underway. The National Institute of Nutrition is preparing new nutrition guidelines for 2011-2020 for submission to the Government in 2010. The guidelines include a package of measures under the heading "Plan of action to accelerate the reduction of stunting (PAARS)" and within this package it is proposed that WIFS should be made available for WRA aged 20-35.

7.2 Lessons learnt

- Close cooperation and open communication between all partners is essential at the national, provincial, district, commune and village levels.
- A compliance survey conducted at an early stage of implementation is beneficial in modifying plans and making timely strategic shifts in project components.

- The supply of IFA and deworming tablets is effective if the time and location of receiving and distributing the supply is standardized and communicated to the implementing team, community members and recipients. However, flexibility in the supply situation must be maintained to ensure poorer or more disadvantaged communities of WRA can be reached.
- The provision of IFA tablets free of cost ensures equitable distribution and higher participation of poorer women, especially ethnic minority groups.
- Blister packaging of IFA tablets is more acceptable than capped bottles. Moreover, the chances of IFA tablets spoiling are reduced with the use of blister packing.
- The production and appropriate packaging of IFA supplements is feasible in a developing country.
- A strong communication strategy is critical for promotion of WIFS and increasing compliance. Counselling by village health workers on the positive benefits of WIFS is critical to increasing compliance. However, the efforts of village health workers need to be complemented by social mobilization and convincing the community of the benefits of WIFS and deworming through print, TV or video clips and local radio.
- Counselling women to consume WIFS on a fixed day facilitates compliance and management of the WIFS programme.
- Monitoring the WIFS intervention and addressing constraints or any adverse effects as soon as possible improves compliance, even in the absence of supervised consumption.

References

1. Casey GJ, *et al*. A free weekly iron-folic acid supplementation and regular deworming programme is associated with improved haemoglobin and iron status indicators in Vietnamese women. *BMC public health*, 2009, 9(1) :261.

2. Mihrshahi S, *et al*. The effectiveness of 4 monthly albendazole treatment in the reduction of soil-transmitted helminth infections in women of reproductive age in Vietnam. *International journal of parasitology*, 2009, 39 (9) 1037-43.

3. Phuc TQ, *et al*. Lessons learned from implementation of a demonstration programme to reduce the burden of anaemia and hookworm in women in Yen Bai province ,Viet Nam. *BMC public health*, 2009, 9(1),266

4. Pasricha SR, *et al*. Anaemia, iron deficiency, meat consumption and hookworm infection in women of reproductive age in Northwest Vietnam. *American Journal of tropical medicine and hygiene*, 87 (3), 2008, pp-375-381.

5. Gerard J. Casey and Beverly Ann Biggs. Personal communications, 18 August 2008 and 15t January 2009.

7.3 Yen Bai Province (Viet Nam) WIFS Programme – A summary

Time framework and coverage	Age group	Anaemia prevalence	Intervention package	Nodal implementing agencies	Impact	Current status
Phase 1 – May 2006, two districts of province covering 50 000 WRA. Phase 2 – March 2008 – to date. Scaled up to the entire province, covering 250 000 WRA.	16-45 years	37.5% WRA (non-pregnant) anaemic and 23.0% iron-deficient.	• WIFS • Albendazole (400 mg) twice a year	• Ministry of Health • Vietnam National Institute of Malariology, Parasitology and Entomology	• Significant decrease in anaemia prevalence from 37.5% to 19.5% – a reduction of 48% in a period of 12 months. • Hookworm infection fell from 76.2% at baseline to 25.2% after 12 months.	• Project scaled up to all districts of the province to reach about 250 000 WRA. • Ministry of Health, Government of Viet Nam is considering scaling up the WIFS programme for WRA to the national level.

Supply and consumption of WIFS

Composition, packaging and supply procurement	Cost	Specific approach used	Specific consumption instructions	IFA Supply to recipients		Supervision during WIFS consumption
				Free / purchased	Access	
Phase 1 – UNICEF supply. IFA tablet contained 60 mg of elemental iron as ferrous sulphate and 0.4 mg of folic acid. Four tablets supplied in double-lidded tamper proof bottles. Phase 2 – Government supply – locally produced by a Viet Nam-based manufacturer (NAPHACO) – changed from bottle to blister packs for IFA tablets. Blister packs designed as six tear-off strips of five tablets per strip.	Cost of WIFS = US$0.40/woman/year	• Fixed-day approach – the decision on which day was left to WRA themselves.	• Consumed on a designated day of the week between meals. • Advised not to take on an empty stomach. • Instructed to swallow tablets with water. • Avoid tea and coffee when taking tablets.	• Free of cost	• Supply channel is well defined up to the the commune health centre (CHS) level. • Village health workers (VHW) collect supply from CHS. • Within the village, distribution to WRA by VHW is on a fixed day. Women are provided with one strip of five tablets per month.	• WIFS not supervised However, Albendazole administration supervised.

Efforts to increase compliance (IEC / Social mobilization / Strategy)

Positive attributes / benefits experienced	Side-effects reported and managed	Supplement-promotion strategy	Compliance
VHW counselled WRA on proven benefits.	Side-effects reported by WRA addressed by health team.	• Promotional activities included use of advocacy and sensitization meetings. Use of TV media, including interviews. • Promotional materials include posters, banners, pictorial handout and timetable for WRA. • Special activities for ensuring high community participation • VHW in charge of counselling. WRA counselled to follow a fixed-day approach. • To increase compliance, the message in the first three months emphasized "healthy women for healthy families". Handouts, posters, calendars for WRA. • Special printed handouts to keep tablets away from children. • Radio programmes, television and video clips.	To increase compliance, WRA are encouraged to take a tablet on a fixed day of the week between meals. Blister packaging and intensified promotional activities to maintain high compliance. Compliance was reported to be about 70% after three months and 69% after 12 months. It was concluded that WRA, if convinced to take WIFS at the start of the project, maintain full compliance.

Training and monitoring

Training	Monitoring Individual cards / registers etc	Other positive contributing factors
• Training of the health team, comprising village, commune and district health workers, was undertaken. Training on causes, treatment and prevention of health risks of anaemia and hookworm infection. Training in administration of WIFS and deworming, management and distribution of supply, monitoring and feedback mechanisms and counselling to address side-effects. • Two manuals developed for trainers and health staff.	• Provincial health authorities monitored supply. Compliance was monitored by a core health team. • In addition, compliance was monitored by an independent NGO.	• Close cooperation and open communication among all partners. • Involvement of an NGO to maintain compliance.

8. Viet Nam (Hai Duong Province)

8.1 Social marketing of weekly iron folic acid supplements (WIFS) - An effective approach for prevention of iron deficiency and anaemia in WRA

PROJECT AT A GLANCE	
Date of programme	• Phase 1 — April 1999 - 2000 • Phase 2 — 2000 onwards
Location	• Hai Duong Province (Viet Nam)
Number of participants	• Estimated 70 000 WRA
Project managed by	• Health sector, in collaboration with Women's Union and Youth Unions
Reduction in anaemia rate	• 56.8% in a nine-month period
Compliance rate	• 92%
Programme costs	• Cost of WIFS = US$0.39 per WRA/year • Cost of WIFS programme = US$5 per WRA/year

A. Project design

Background

Viet Nam has about 20 million women of reproductive age (WRA). Iron deficiency and iron deficiency anaemia are public health problems in the country. The programme for anaemia control is focused on the provision of daily IFA tablets to pregnant women from the first antenatal visit. However, despite this policy, the prevalence of anaemia among pregnant women, according to a survey in 1999, remains high and is estimated to be over 50%. It was therefore considered important to address this problem by reaching women prior to pregnancy by introducing preventive measures.

Target group

A trial project was launched in two phases by the National Institute of Nutrition, with the support of the WHO Regional Office for the Western Pacific. In Phase 1, covering the period April 1999 to December 2000, the Thanh Mien district of Hai Duong Province was covered. The district has 19 rural communes and a population of 135 000. One quarter of the population (34 000) was estimated to be WRA. In Phase 2, based on the results of Phase 1, the trial project was continued in the Thanh Mien district and extended to an additional district, Binh Giang, in the same province.

Project objectives

The three specific objectives of the pilot project were:

- to introduce a new preventive supplementation approach, using WIFS for WRA, promoted through social marketing and mobilization activities;
- to assess the effectiveness of such a combined approach in improving knowledge, attitudes, and practices regarding the prevention and control of IDA; and
- to define the duration of pre-pregnancy, preventive IFA supplementation needed to have a significant impact on haemoglobin and iron status.

> The programme for anaemia control is focused on the provision of daily IFA tablets to pregnant women from the first antenatal visit. However, despite this policy, the prevalence of anaemia among pregnant women, according to a survey in 1999, remains high, at an estimate of over 50%.

The project therefore aimed to assess the effectiveness of the WIFS approach under the usual non-supervised programme conditions, but with the introduction of well-designed community-based social mobilization and social marketing initiatives.

Project roles and responsibilities

The health sector was the nodal department in charge of the project, since both curative and preventive health activities are the responsibilities of this sector at district, commune and village levels. Each commune has a health centre staffed by four to six health workers. Additionally, each village has one village health worker. Besides the health network, the various other community organizations in the district, such as the Youth Union, Women's Union, Farmers Association and Veteran's Association, also participated in project activities. The Women's Union, a well organized network linking district headquarters with communes and villages, participated actively as collaborators in health care programmes and in social mobilization activities. These collaborators, in the first phase of implementation, received money as incentives from sales of supplements, as described below, through the social marketing approach.

District- and commune-level organizational support was strengthened to improve project management. District and commune steering committees were formed, comprising representatives from the Health Office, the Women's Union and the Committee for Protection and Care of Children (CPCC), and from other sectors such as education, information and culture. The function of these steering committees was to provide overall management support and policy guidance for development and modification of operational plans and their implementation. Monthly meetings were organized to discuss progress and resolve issues.

B. *Process and progress*

Training

Two-day training sessions were conducted for about 811 persons, including health staff, members of the steering committees, about 100 high-school teachers and 570 Women's Union network members from district to commune levels. Training sessions used a participatory approach and focused on information on anaemia and prenatal and postnatal care, as well as on imparting skills for effective communication, organization of training sessions, monitoring of sales, use of IFA supplements and management of funds.

In the case of teachers, training content focused on the importance of preventing anaemia in adolescent girls and measures for the prevention of iron deficiency, including the importance of WIFS. In addition, a special effort was made to impart communication skills to teachers.

IFA supply

Social marketing of the product was central to the strategy of the trial project. A fixed-day approach was used for promoting WIFS. IFA tablets were produced especially for the phase 1 project by UNILAB (Manila), as per the WHO-recommended formula. The tablets for non-pregnant WRA were pink in colour and each contained 60 mg of elemental iron and 3.5mg of folic acid. The tablets for pregnant mothers were red and each contained 120 mg of elemental iron and 3.5mg of folic acid. WRA who were reported to be pregnant were switched to a weekly intake of supplements with the higher iron concentration. A systematic effort was also made to compare this weekly unsupervised consumption of IFA by pregnant mothers with the ongoing programme of giving daily IFA from the first antenatal visit onwards. The tablets were in foil packaging to ensure stability and protection. Each package contained four tablets, or a month's supply.

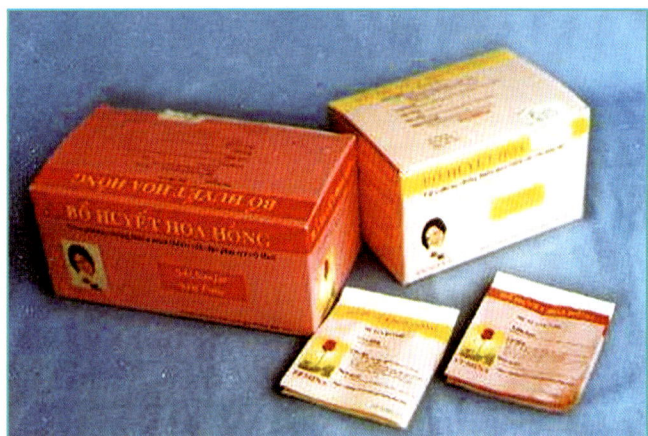

IFA Supplement packaging in Viet Nam

It was considered critical to give the IFA supplements a new image. Following a rapid formative assessment, IFA was given a new name and a positive image and the tablets were packed in attractive packs. The name chosen for the iron supplement was Bo Huyet Hoa Hong (BHHH) meaning "nutrition supplement for healthy blood". A logo for the product was designed, featuring a picture of a beautiful girl holding a rose. The inclusion of a rose suggested an association between the consumption of IFA supplements and a healthy blood supply, resulting in attractiveness. Along with the logo, the following message was standardized in the local language "take one BHHH only once a week — you will feel beautiful and healthy". This message, along with the logo, was printed on packs and used in all the IEC materials ranging from posters to billboards, banners, promotional cars and loudspeakers, to give a new image to iron supplements. All these efforts were directed at shifting the public's perception from viewing the IFA supplement as medicine to seeing it as a protector of health, "good" blood and beauty.

Efforts were directed at shifting the public's perception from viewing the IFA supplement as medicine to seeing it as a protector of health, "good" blood and beauty.

To promote the supplements among non-pregnant WRA, the Women's Union network was made responsible for selling the tablets and motivating the women in their own communes. These women, being from the local community, could easily communicate with WRA and educate non-pregnant women to regularly purchase and consume the supplements. Compared with health personnel, these local women were particularly effective promoters and were well-accepted by WRA in their communities. Initially, WIFS was made available to high-school girls through their mothers or sisters. However, in the second phase, the supplements were provided to adolescent girls through the school system.

Cost

The price of tablets was fixed following in-depth interviews with local women and family members. A subsidized price of 1000 Vietnamese dong (VDN) or

US$0.08 per blister pack containing a month's supply of four tablets was found to be affordable. The cost of a yearly supply per person was thus estimated to be about 12 000 VDN or US$0.96. The cost per blister pack was decided in consultation with rural women and families, and it was agreed by them that money generated from the sale of supplements should be used to partially meet the operational cost of the trial project as follows:

- 20% for payment to women collaborators;
- 30% for meeting the cost of management and regular communication; and
- 50% as a bank deposit for a revolving fund to buy new supplements, managed by the district steering committee.

The steering committee was responsible for implementing the operational plan and consisted of representatives from the district health office and the Women's Union, and from the education, information and culture sectors. It should be noted, however, that pregnant women received IFA supplements for daily consumption free of charge from government health staff, following the local policy for daily IFA supplements.

IEC activities

For effective community mobilization, project-communication activities were built into the monthly agenda of the Women's Union. The members of the Women's Union organized monthly sessions with WRA on the importance of WIFS. The sessions were made interesting through the use of drama, poems and folk songs, with content related to the project. Competitions were also organized. Additionally, teachers in high schools were trained to impart information to high-school, adolescent girls and community involvement was ensured through other organizations, including the Elder's Club, the Veteran's Organization and the Youth Organization in each commune. Promotional activities included campaigns to motivate WRA to buy and use weekly supplements, and ensured community participation by generating interest and motivating the community to be partners in the care of WRA. For the campaigns, banners were hung on main roads and communication cars moved around villages to raise awareness of anaemia prevention and motivate the purchase and consumption of WIFS. A booklet on preventing anaemia was distributed to communities (WRA and their families), and information was also communicated through the local radio station. High schools organized essay-writing competitions on the subject of "Preventing iron deficiency anaemia".

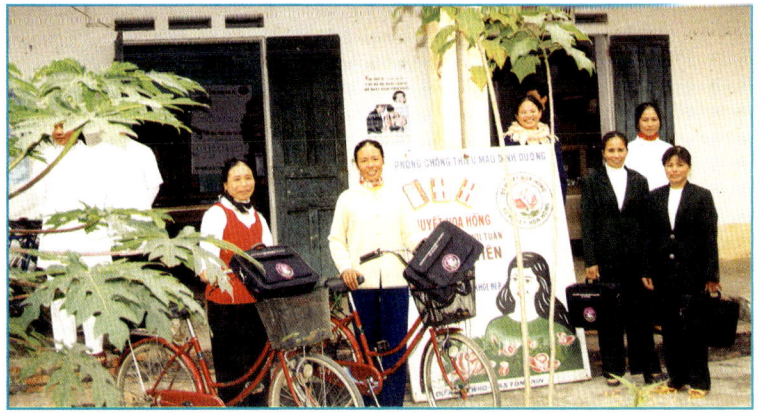

Billboard at health station

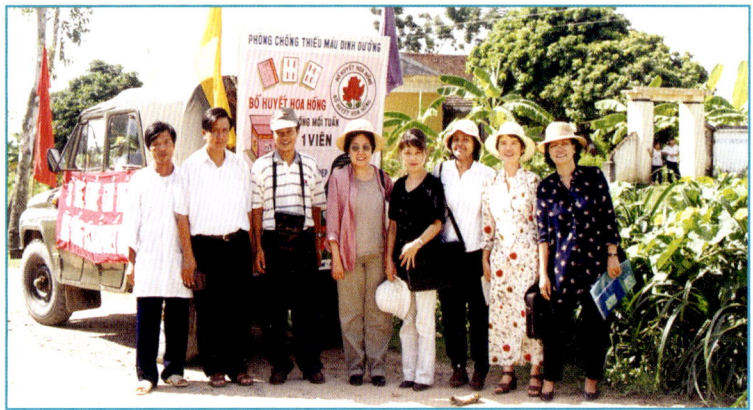
Project team and promotional vehicle

Two advocacy meetings were organized, one for representatives of various ministries to seek their consensus and ensure a supportive policy environment, and the second with the project implementers at the district and commune levels to seek their consensus and commitment.

To sustain interest and support, a continuous dialogue was maintained between the project team and community leaders. The rates of purchase and consumption of WIFS was noted by commune members in special record books. Information on sales and consumption of WIFS was reviewed every three months and actions were taken to streamline money management and ensure reported problems were quickly resolved. Moreover, reports of drops in sales of IFA supplements were immediately addressed by organizing impromptu workshops with community and Women's Union leaders, and by launching a campaign to reinforce the message on regular consumption of the weekly supplements. Such actions helped to check any decline in purchase, as was evident from the increase in sales observed after the decline at nine months: sales rose to 92% in the first six months, then dropped to around 65% at around nine months and rose again to about 80% at 12 months. Consumption was not supervised. However, all women who bought the supplements reported that they consumed them regularly.

Phase 2

In both districts of Phase 1 and 2, non-pregnant women were motivated to buy and consume WIFS. However, the strategy in Phase 2 differed from Phase 1 with regard to the following:

1. In Phase 2, the composition of the supplements was changed to conform to the national Government's approved formulation. Each tablet contained the same amount of iron, but 0.4 mg instead of 3.5 mg of folic acid. The supplements were produced locally by the Medical Scientific Technology Centre, Hanoi Medical University, and were packed in blisters of 30 tablets, instead of the four-tablet packs used in Phase 1. The cost was almost one third that in the first phase — 2500 VDN or US $0.20 for 30 tablets (a seven-month supply) compared with 1000 VDN or US $0.08 for four tablets (a one-month supply) in Phase 1.

2. Funds generated from the sale of supplements in Phase 1 were used to meet the cost of purchasing new supplements for the second phase.

IFA supplements were stored at commune health stations and in local private pharmacies.

3. In Phase 2, commune members or members of women's clubs were given no financial incentives for promoting and selling supplements in communes and schools.

4. Adolescent girls were reached through schools, unlike in Phase 1 where mothers and sisters handed IFA supplements to high-school girls. School activities were noted to be a very important part of community mobilization. Preliminary results indicated a higher compliance rate in Phase 1 than in Phase 2.

Evaluation

In Phase 1, the impact of WIFS was studied against the baseline information after a period of 4.5, 9 and 12 months. Four aspects of change were studied: changes in knowledge, attitudes and practices; compliance in taking supplements; prevalence of side-effects; and laboratory assessment of iron status.

The findings revealed that, in Phase1, the sale of WIFS continued to increase, with the rate of buying and using supplements increasing from about 54% to 92% over a period of six months. There was then a decline to less than 70% by the ninth month. However, following a special campaign, there was an increase in sales. Interestingly, the reported side-effects associated with consumption of tablets by non-pregnant WRA decreased with time (Figure 14).

Figure 14: Side-effects of taking weekly IFA supplements in non-pregnant women of reproductive age

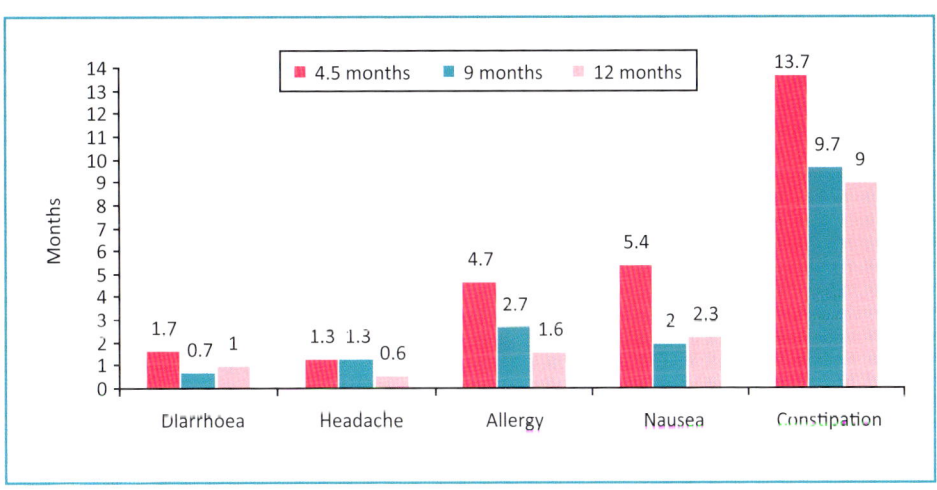

With consumption of WIFS, positive benefits were reported, such as feeling stronger and less tired, as well as experiencing an increase in appetite and improved sleep patterns (Figure 15).

Figure 15: Perception of impact of WIFS in non-pregnant women

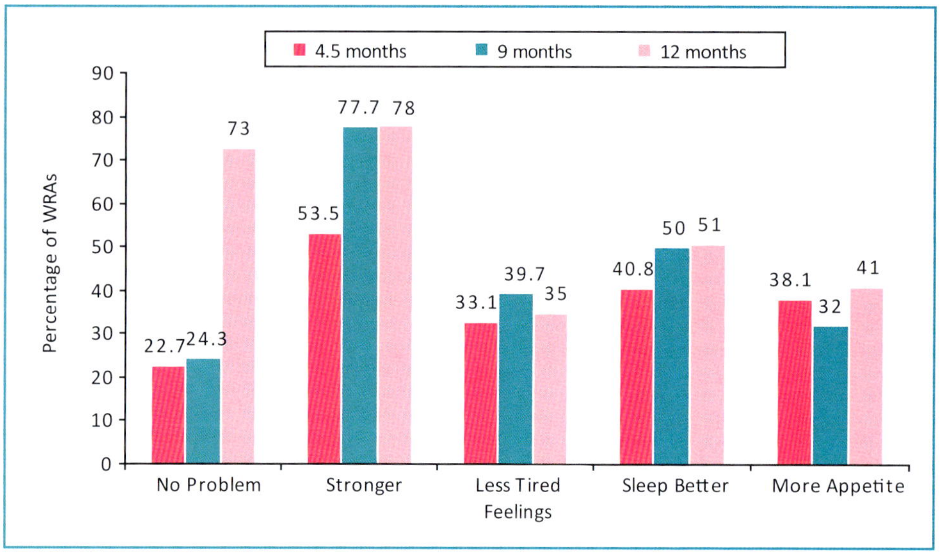

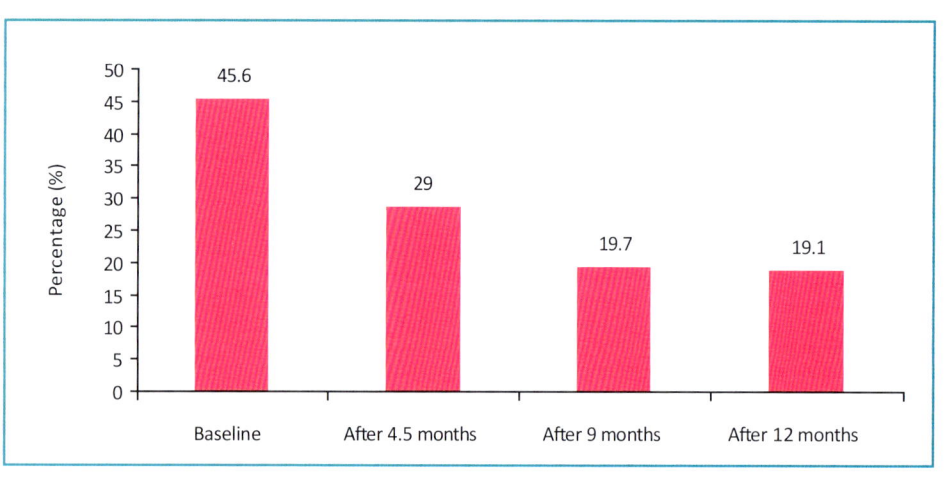

The impact of WIFS on haemoglobin and serum ferritin concentration was evident, despite the fact that consumption was not supervised. There was a decrease in anaemia prevalence from 45.6% at baseline to 19.7% after nine months of project implementation (Figure 16).

Figure 16: Anaemia prevalence at each visit in non-pregnant women (weekly group)

By the third month of the expansion phase, in 2003, over 50% of WRA were reported to be buying and using IFA supplements in the two intervention districts (Figure 17). However, since the IFA supplements in phase 2 were less attractive, due to fewer social marketing activities and no financial incentives being used to promote and sell supplements in communes and schools, greater efforts were needed to encourage and motivate WRA to regularly buy and use WIFS.

Figure 17: Buying and using IFA supplements by non-pregnant women in the two intervention districts in Viet Nam in 2003

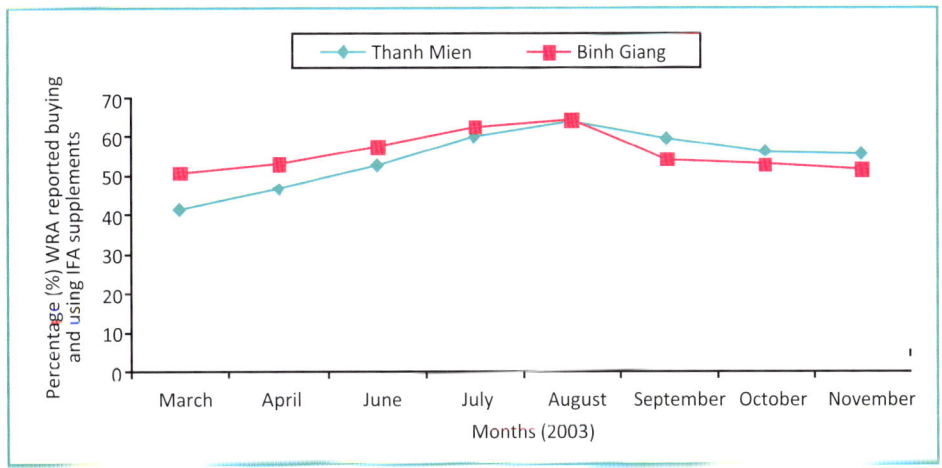

One very significant finding of the project was that WIFS, when taken three to six months before the beginning of pregnancy and continued regularly during pregnancy, with a higher weekly dose of iron, resulted in good iron stores and improved haemoglobin during the first and second trimesters of pregnancy. Moreover, the prevalence of low birth weight was lowest among women supplemented weekly during pregnancy.

8.2 Lessons learnt

- Intervention with WIFS, irrespective of supervision, is effective in reducing anaemia in WRA.

- Prevention of iron deficiency prior to the onset of pregnancy is critical to prepare for safe motherhood. Therefore, for prevention of anaemia it is crucial to provide WIFS to adolescent girls through the school system.

- Implementing a well-designed, community-based social mobilization and social marketing approach is effective in increasing demand, purchase and regular intake of WIFS by WRA in rural communities, even without a proper marketing system through health services.

- For effective social mobilization, involvement of non-health sectors is critical. Additionally, strong support and commitment by local authorities and active community participation are crucial to the success of community-based health and nutrition programmes.

- Linking district health centres to non-health systems, such as women's groups or communes, is effective in managing the logistics of IFA supplement distribution. Women's Union collaborators can play a central role in the logistical management of supplements, since this network of women is well-informed of the local situation and better equipped to convince WRA to consume WIFS as a preventive measure and not as a cure.

- Supplying the IFA tablets attractively packaged and at a fixed price is important for success in social marketing. Fixing the price in consultation with WRA is helpful in ensuring acceptance of the agreed price.

- The country's capacity to produce IFA supplements should be assessed to ensure the provision of a good quality local product, at an affordable price.
- A new name and a positive image increases acceptance of IFA, as well as demand and consumption. A distinct, attractive logo, which further highlights the association of IFA tablets with health and beauty, increases the value of IFA tablets for WRA and helps to achieve a shift in viewing WIFS, not as medicine, but as a long-term strategy for protection of health and beauty.
- Use of a fixed-day approach facilitates the management of WIFS programmes.

- An effective IEC strategy maintains a high level of motivation to purchase and consume IFA, even in the absence of supervision during consumption.
- Positive benefits are evident, while side-effects are rare. Interestingly, side-effects decrease with time of usage of WIFS.
- It is important to organize regular promotional reinforcement activities to counteract any negative influences and to address any decrease in sales of IFA tablets. In special situations, such as harvest seasons, modifications in strategy are required to help busy women remember to take their tablets. Communication strategies need to be modified and stepped up in special situations.

- Participatory training sessions are effective, not only for imparting technical information on anaemia, but for development of skills in effective communication, monitoring of sales and use of IFA supplements, as well as in the management of logistics and funds.
- Monitoring of sales is feasible with the active involvement of commune members. Special recording registers are useful for recording and monitoring sales.

References

1. Khan NC, *et al*. Community mobilization and social marketing to promote weekly iron folic acid supplementation: a new approach toward controlling anaemia among women of reproductive age in Vietnam. *Nutrition reviews*, December 2005, 63 (12): S87-S94.

2. Berger J, *et al*. Community mobilization and social marketing to promote weekly iron folic acid supplementation in women of reproductive age in Vietnam: impact on anaemia and iron status *Nutrition reviews,* December 2005, 63 (12): S95-S108.

3. Report on carrying out phase 2 of weekly iron folate supplement for WRA to control anaemia.

8.3 Hai Duong Province (Viet Nam) WIFS Programme – A summary

Time framework and coverage	Age group	Anaemia prevalence	Intervention package	Nodal implementing agencies	Impact	Current status
• Phase 1 – April 1999-2000, one district of province, WRA population (25%) = 34 000 • Phase 2 – phase 1 continued and an additional district of the province included. Total WRA population almost 70 000	Not defined	Anaemia among WRA 45.6% and among pregnant women over 50%.	• WIFS	• Health sector, in collaboration with Women's Union, Youth Union.	• Anaemia prevalence decreased from 45.6% at baseline to 19.7% after nine months – 56.8% decrease. • WIFS taken three to six months prior to pregnancy and continued during pregnancy with a higher dose resulted in good iron stores and improved haemoglobin during the first and second trimester.	• This project served as a basis for the expansion of WIFS for WRA to another district and for the introduction of WIFS for WRA in Yen Bai province. WIFS for WRA is one of the approaches included in the Plan of Action for the Acceleration of the Reduction of Stunting (PAARS) in Viet Nam.

Supply and consumption of WIFS

Composition, packaging and supply procurement	Cost	Specific approach used	Specific consumption instructions	FA Supply to recipients		Supervision during WIFS consumption
				Free / purchased	Access	
Phase 1 – UNILAB produced IFA tablets for weekly dose to non-pregnant women were pink in colour and contained 60 mg of elemental iron and 3.5 mg of folic acid. IFA tablets for weekly dose to pregnant mothers were red in colour and contained 120 mg of elemental iron and 3.5 mg of folic acid. Foil packaging of four tablets – one month's supply. Attractive packs. Phase 2– produced by Medical Science Technology Centre, composition changed to government policy norms, containing 60 mg of elemental iron and 0.4 mg of folic acid in blister packs of 30 tablets.	Phase 1 – subsidized price US$0.08 for a blister pack of four IFA tablets. Price was decided in consultation with rural WRA and families. Cost / beneficiary for pilot project ** Phase 2 – Government new package and cost significantly less – US $ 0.20** for 30 tablets or US$0.03 for 4 tablets or US$ 0.39 for 52 weeks.	• Fixed-day approach. • Specific day decided in consultation with local population.	Take supplement at night before sleeping.	• WRAs, including high-school girls purchased WIFS. • Pregnant women received WIFS free of charge.	• Women's Union network motivated and sold supplements to WRA local community. • In Phase 1 mothers and sisters purchased WIFS for high-school girls in the family. In phase 2, schoolgirls purchased WIFS from teachers. • Pregnant women received WIFS (free) from health workers.	Not supervised

**Cost estimated for 30 000 WRA covered at the cost of US $ 150 000 (excludes cost of IFA tablets) = US$5/woman covered by the project

Efforts to increase compliance (IEC / Social mobilization / Strategy)

Positive attributes / benefits experienced	Side-effects reported and managed	Supplement-promotion strategy	Compliance
Feeling stronger, less tired, increased appetite, sleeping better.	Diarrhoea, headache, allergy, nausea and constipation. Side-effects decreased with time.	• Social marketing and mobilization activities included. • A new positive image for product. Name of supplement – BHHH in local language (meaning nutrition supplement for healthy blood). • Logo for the product – a picture of a beautiful girl holding a rose. Associating IFA with healthy blood, resulting in attractiveness. • Shift IFA from "medicine" to "good" blood and beauty. • Message – "beauty and health". • Logo printed on all IEC materials – bills, billboards, banners, promotional cars and loudspeakers, booklets. • Social mobilization – monthly sessions in women's clubs, teachers in high schools, other youth groups. Drama, poems and folk songs related to the programme. • Campaign activities in schools and organizations, etc. • Note – Phase 2 – package less attractive and greater effort required.	Higher compliance in phase 1 than phase 2. Sales rose to 92% in first six months and 80% at 12 months. In phase 2, after nine months, compliance varied from 42% to 65%. Reduction in compliance was attributed to WIFS being less attractive in presentation, fewer social marketing activities and no financial incentives to promote and sell supplements.

Training and monitoring

Training	Monitoring Individual cards / registers etc	Other positive contributing factors
• Training (two days) for health staff ranging from district to commune level, high-school teachers. • Training, using participatory approach, focused on information on anaemia, prenatal and postnatal care, as well as imparting skills for effective education and communication, organization of training sessions, and monitoring of sale and usage of IFA supplements, as well as management of funds. For teachers, additional relevant technical information on anaemia and its prevention was included in the training.	• Commune members recorded information on sales and consumption in special recording registers. Reviewed information every three months for programme implementation.	• High-level advocacy meetings organized for two ministries (health and education) and their consensus sought. • District- and commune-level steering committees for management and support – monthly meetings. • In phase 1, sales were noted to be better than in phase 2 since women received monetary incentives.

9. Cambodia

9.1 WIFS Programme for girls in secondary schools and WRA in rural communities and factories

PROJECT AT A GLANCE	
Date of programme	• Phase 1 – March 2001 – December 2002 • Phase 2 – December 2002 –2008 • Phase 3 – 2008 - Present
Location	• Phnom Penh and Kampong Speu Province
Number of participants	• Estimated 113 000 (78 000 schoolgirls, 33 000 WRA in factories and communities)
Project managed by	• Cambodian Ministry of Health
Reduction in anaemia rate	• Haemoglobin levels increased significantly more in schoolgirls who took WIFS (+ 3.6 g/l) than in schoolgirls who did not (+0.8g/l) over a six-month period
Compliance rate	• 71% WRA in communities • 57% WRA in factories • 55% schoolgirls • 43.8% - 57.4% WRA in rural villages
Programme costs	• Cost of WIFS programme = US$5 per WRA/year

A. Project design

Target group

Anaemia is a serious public health problem in Cambodia, with 57% of pregnant women and 47% of WRA reported to be anaemic by the Cambodia Demographic and Health Surveys 2005.

Anaemia is a serious public health problem in Cambodia, with 57% of pregnant women and 47% of WRA reported to be anaemic by the Cambodia Demographic and Health Surveys 2005. In order to help reduce the rates of anaemia in WRA, a new approach was introduced through a pilot programme in 2001-2002. The project aimed to replenish iron stores before women became pregnant, using WIFS. The programme was implemented in seven garment factories in and around Phnom Penh and in 139 rural villages and five secondary schools in Kampong Speu Province. A total of 24 000 women were reached in the project, conducted between March 2001 and December 2002.

Programme objectives

The objectives of the programme were:

- to introduce, under programme conditions and through the application of a social marketing and participatory-communication approach, a preventive WIFS programme for non-pregnant WRA in selected garment factories, secondary schools and rural communities;

- to assess the effectiveness of the WIFS programme in improving the knowledge, attitudes and practices, as well as haemoglobin levels, of non-pregnant WRA in all three target areas; and

- to assess the effects of deworming, combined with IFA supplementation, on haemoglobin levels in subgroups of selected women in each of the three project target areas.

Programme roles and responsibilities

The nodal implementing agency was the National Nutrition Programme (NNP) of the National Maternal and Child Health Centre (NMCHC), Cambodian Ministry of Health. The project was implemented in collaboration with WHO, UNICEF and the Japanese Government, who provided substantial funding. A National Programme Steering Committee was established. Stakeholders included the Ministry of Health, NMCHC, WHO, UNICEF, other sectors and NGOs working in the health sector.

B. Process and progress

Implementing the WIFS programme in factories

A separate strategy was developed to implement WIFS in factories. The Occupational Health Department was in charge of selecting factories in collaboration with the National Maternal and Child Health Centre. A total of 10 459 women were covered in seven factories.

The strategy was based on the principle of social marketing of IFA tablets to promote weekly consumption. To achieve the objectives of the programme, an effort was made to:

- ensure a timely and continuous supply of IFA;
- establish a system to make the supplements available to women;
- create demand for supplements through an effective social mobilization strategy;
- provide training for effective implementation; and
- develop a system for monitoring supplement sales, compliance and consumption.

For social marketing of the IFA supplements, developing an attractive name and image was considered crucial. The name "Red Rose", which in the local language is *Kolap Krahorm* or *KK*, was selected. Red Rose was considered the most suitable name since it portrayed an image of women "glowing with good health". Dialogue with the community also indicated that women associated roses with beauty, good health, a glowing complexion and a positive self-image. Moreover, beauty was also related to freedom from fatigue and tiredness during the menstruation period. The name Red Rose was, therefore, considered the most suitable to generate a positive attitude towards consumption of IFA. The National Centre for Health Promotion (NCHP) designed the logo, which showed a beautiful Apsara (fairy) holding a red rose. The logo was displayed on all IEC materials as well as on the packaging of IFA supplements.

> For social marketing of the IFA supplements, developing an attractive name and image was considered crucial.

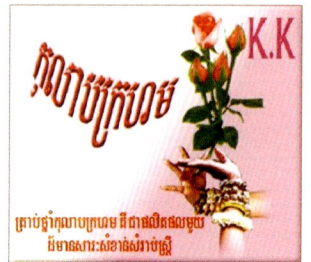 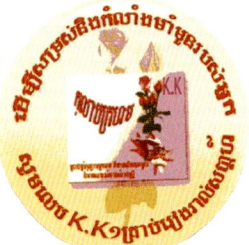

Logo and cover of WIFS packaging in Cambodia

IFA supply and IEC activities (factories)

The IFA tablets, containing 60 mg of elemental iron and 3.5 mg of folic acid, were produced in an elliptical shape, with a film coating for ease of swallowing. Packaging was made attractive in the form of blister packs of four tablets and tertiary packs containing 50 small packs. The WHO Regional Office for the Western Pacific procured the supply from United Laboratories Inc, Manila, Philippines. The blister and tertiary packaging was done by the national packing station of the Ministry of Health, situated in Phnom Penh, with funding from WHO. The specially designed logo, along with a standardized message and the price of the product (established in consultation with the community), was printed on the IFA packages, as well as on all IEC materials, including posters, stickers and leaflets. These IEC materials (examples presented below) also contained information on anaemia prevention, the use of iron-rich foods and the importance of weekly consumption of the Red Rose IFA supplement.

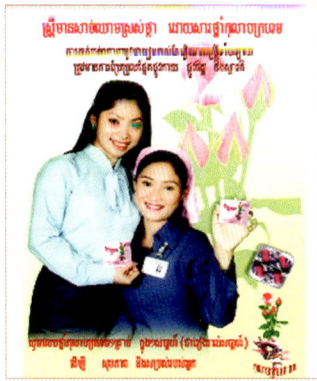
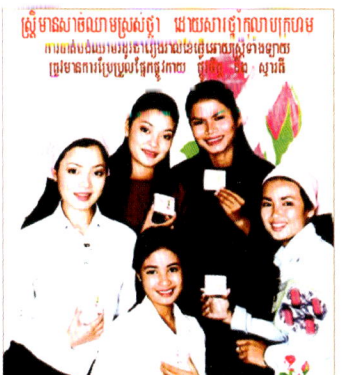
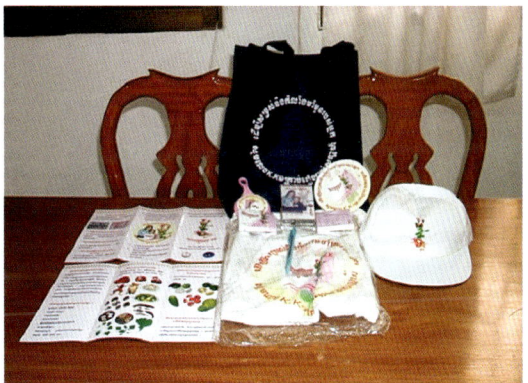

Posters, leaflets and other materials used for IEC activities

To promote the product, additional materials, such as billboards, hats, tee-shirts, shoulder bags for secondary-school girls and mirrors, were produced with the logo and key message printed on them. A part of the profit derived from WIFS was used as incentives for those selling the supplements and to set up a revolving fund to purchase additional supplements.

In each of the seven factories, team leaders were selected for each group of 20-50 women. These leaders were in charge of distributing the IFA supplement to women in their groups once a month. IFA supplements in factories, as per labour policy, were supplied without any charge. The supply was replenished every month during monitoring visits by staff from the nodal agency, NMCHC. Team leaders organized distribution to women in factories during working hours. The team leaders maintained a record of the number of IFA tablets distributed. During the first three months of the programme, team leaders were also in charge of imparting information on the benefits of WIFS and informing women of the importance of consuming foods rich in iron and other nutrients, and a mobile team of three to six members organized education sessions on Sundays, the factory workers' day off.

A fixed-day approach was institutionalized for promoting and ensuring the supply and consumption of WIFS. Every Saturday of the month was fixed for consuming supplements. On Saturday evenings, women were reminded to consume their IFA tablets at night, before sleeping.

A programme launch was organized to create excitement and interest in WIFS among stakeholders. Cambodian media provided good coverage of the launch in each factory on the national television network. The event was held on Saturday so that the factory workers were not disrupted and a higher level of participation was ensured. Special education campaigns focusing on the benefits of WIFS and the positive results experienced by women in the first two months of the programme resulted in overcoming rumours. Rumours included that the IFA tablets were: amphetamine tablets to make women work harder, family planning pills or infertility pills, and weight-increasing drugs.

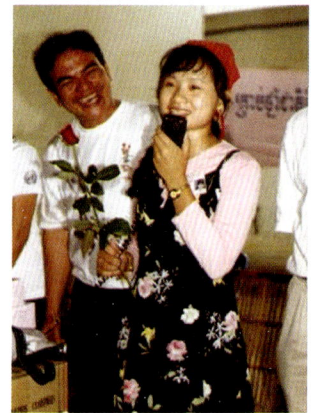

Woman taking part in a special campaign held in factories

Training (factories)

The team leaders in factories were trained in counselling and peer education. These team leaders, along with three to six people from each of the factories, were also responsible for organizing mobile team educational activities for the factory women on Sundays. The NMCHC team of two people conducted monitoring in factories every month for the first three months, and then every two months. A standardized monitoring form was used to facilitate analysis and feedback.

Implementing the WIFS programme in communities

The WIFS programme for WRA in communities, including adolescents, was implemented by integrating it with the ongoing UNICEF-supported Community Action for Social Development (CASD) programme. CASD had been launched in 1996 and later implemented as a children's-rights programme (or Seth Kuma Programme or SKP) from 2002, in six provinces, covering 1130 villages, 120 communes, and 18 districts. The programme had the following major components: capacity-building; community education and child care; water, sanitation and environment; health, hygiene and nutrition; protection and care of vulnerable women and children; and credit, employment and income. The WIFS project formed an operational link with SKP by integrating it with ongoing SKP activities.

IFA supply and IEC activities (communities)

The first province selected for this integration was Kampong Speu. In 2002, WIFS was implemented in the SKP programme area, covering five of the 18 districts, 22 of the 89 communes and 371 of the 1331 villages. An action plan was developed in a two-day workshop, with the participation of district SKP staff, as well as MCH staff and staff of the school health programme. Promotion, counselling and the sale of IFA was undertaken by a key community person, such as a village or a commune leader, or a village development community member, and by a team of two peer educators per village. The latter were often women, well known in their village and in charge of health activities in the village development committees.

The adolescent girls of the community, to a great extent, were reached through the school network. A fixed-day strategy was used. Peer educators (two schoolgirls with leadership abilities) and teachers (one teacher from each of the target classes) were responsible for supplying the supplements. Supplements were sold to schoolchildren for US$0.10 per blister pack of four tablets, a monthly supply. Teachers also monitored consumption of WIFS and maintained records of sale and consumption. The role of peer educators was to promote WIFS as a preventive supplement and to disseminate information on nutrition and iron-rich foods. These educators were also viewed as role models who would inspire women to be more pro-active in improving their health. A school WIFS committee of teachers and students was formed to manage funds from the sale of WIFS through a school fund. The school system provided a highly supportive environment for imparting knowledge and influencing behavioural practices to control and prevent anaemia. Informing adolescent girls of their haemoglobin levels further motivated them to take WIFS.

Activities

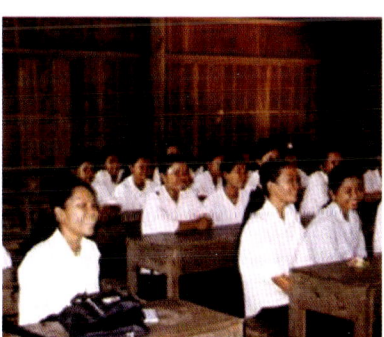
In classroom

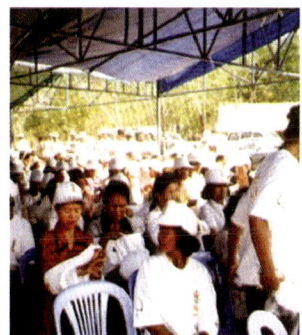
Launching at community

In some villages, WIFS were sold centrally, following a regular monthly village meeting, while in other villages the peer educator went from door to door promoting and selling WIFS. The tablets were priced, in consultation with the community, at US$ 0.10 (400 Riel) for a blister pack of four tablets. Of the money paid, 75% was set aside for the village's revolving fund to generate further income, while 25% was allocated as an incentive for the seller of the supplement. The price was kept uniform for schoolgirls and village women. However, women listed as being poor by the village development committees were not charged for the supplements. Peer educators, in Commune Development Committee meetings, reviewed WIFS sales and ordered supplies for subsequent months. Based on this information, packs of IFA supplements were supplied to the peer educators by the SKP commune team. The central medical store provided the WIFS supply through the health system network at the commune and provincial levels.

Two special events were organized to launch the product: a small launch for a cluster of schools and a big launch for schools and the community in January 2002. The SKP provincial team, with the support of the MCH department, organized the launch. The major launch, in Kampong Speu, was attended by over 800 women from the neighbouring village of Wat Phnom (Samrong Torang district), provincial- and national-level leaders and politicians, and influential monks. In addition, a lottery was announced and held after the first five months of the programme to help maintain interest and excitement. The event was covered on television and in the newspaper.

Monitoring (communities)

A monitoring system was established by NMCHC in the first three months of the project and monitoring activities were undertaken every three months by the SKP team. The standardized monitoring format prepared included information on: time of receipt of the IFA supply, the number and percentage of women buying the supplement in target areas, and the number reporting side-effects. Reports of rumours associated with IFA usage, the number of women discontinuing use of IFA supplements, reasons for discontinuation, timely delivery of the supplements, the amount of money generated for the revolving fund and the use of the revolving fund were also monitored. Information was recorded on a monitoring form every three months, at village, commune, district and provincial levels. In the first three months, the monitoring task was undertaken in collaboration with the NMCHC. The monitoring reports, however, were sent to the national level NMCHC programme team for the entirety of the project.

Training (communities)

The key commune persons and peer educators of 139 villages, as well as schoolteachers, were trained in a two-day session on the WIFS programme, promotion and sales of IFA supplements, recording of information on monitoring forms, and counselling on WIFS and nutrition education. The training also focused on in-putting funds, generated from the sale of WIFS, into the existing village revolving funds. Key trainers from SKP conducted the training. All participants were provided with a manual on the WIFS project, as well as a sample pack of supplements, a poster, a sticker and a programme tee-shirt. The NMCHC staff of the Ministry of Health supervised training at the commune level.

Evaluation

The impact of WIFS was studied seven months after the launch, in December 2001. Women consuming supplements reported positive results: sleeping better (73%), increased appetite (62%) and feeling stronger (42%); while negative effects reported included black faeces (39%), headaches (9%), diarrhoea (4%) and nausea

(4%). Compliance was reported to vary in different set-ups, from 71% among rural women to 57% in female factory workers and 55% in schoolgirls.

The mean increase in haemoglobin levels over six months was reported to be significantly higher for Cambodian adolescent girls who took WIFS than for those who did not take the supplements, 3.6 g/L compared to 0.8 g/L.

The impact on haemoglobin was also studied in garment factory workers. Baseline data was collected for 1181 garment factory workers (median age = 21 years), but final data analysis after follow-up was possible for only 478 workers. Data revealed that workers belonging to the group with more education (completed grades 11 or 12) showed a mean elevation in haemoglobin of 7.4 g/L, greater than that of the least educated group (Table 14). The difference was statistically significant.

Table 14: Multivariate linear regression model* for women working in garment factories in Cambodia participating in a WIFS programme

Highest school grade attained	Change in Hb level [#]	P
11 – 12	7.4 g/L	0.04
9 – 10	1.4 g/L	0.48
7 – 8	1.1 g/L	0.46
5 – 6	0.5 g/L	0.72
4 or lower (reference group)	n/a	n/a

*The model was adjusted for potential confounding by these variables: initial Hb levels, age, salary and body mass index (all in quartiles), having fever during the two weeks prior to baseline (binary) and having diarrhoea 24 hours prior to baseline (binary).
[#] Above that of the reference group.

Similarly, the impact of WIFS on rural women was evident. A total of 1021 rural village women (median age = 32 years) were enrolled at the time of the baseline survey, while final haemoglobin levels were studied six months later in only 638 women. A total of 383 women were not included in the evaluation because they were either not available for the follow-up study or were pregnant. Women of lower socioeconomic status also had low initial mean haemoglobin levels of 116 g/L, compared with 120g/L for the higher socioeconomic group. Rural village women belonging to the "high" socioeconomic group reported better compliance in taking the IFA supplements, 57.4%, versus 43.8% in the "low" socioeconomic group.

Table 15: Socioeconomic status (SES) groups stratified by participant reported usage of WIFS at follow up for rural village women in Cambodia (N=638)

Socioeconomic status	Taking WIFS	Not taking WIFS
High (N=94)	57.4%	42.6%
Middle (N=416)	49.3%	50.7%
Low (N=128)	43.8%	56.3%

* Chi-squared P for linear trend = 0.046

It was evident that women who were better off socioeconomically were more accepting of the WIFS programme, despite the fact that no fees were charged to the poorest rural village women. The findings indicate that the WIFS programme, for women in the lower socioeconomic group, could be improved by re-designing the communication strategy.

Scaling up

Following the demonstration project, an expanded WIFS programme was planned in 2005 but, due to delay in receipt of IFA supplements, was implemented after a period of three years, in 2008. All 240 secondary schools of five provinces (Kep, Kampot, Kampong Speu, Pursat and Kampong Thom) were covered through the school system, while WRA living in rural communities in one operational district in Kampong Thom (Baray Santouk) were covered through the health system. From January to November 2008, approximately 60 000 schoolgirls and 33 000 WRA were enrolled in the programme. WIFS containing 60 mg of iron and 3.5 mg of folic acid were provided free of cost in the expansion programme, along with weekly health and nutrition education by schoolteachers to adolescent girls in school and education by health staff to WRA once a month. Unlike the pilot project, the schoolgirls and WRA in the expansion programme received WIFS free of cost. Education sessions included topics on the causes, effects, prevention and control of anaemia; the importance of WIFS; iron-rich foods; and the side-effects of WIFS. Following evaluation, a scaling-up programme was planned to launch the National Policy for Anaemia Prevention and Control in 2010. Due to limited funding for social marketing, the Ministry of Health decided, in 2008, to distribute WIFS free of charge. However, a social marketing strategy is being considered as one of the strategies for the distribution of WIFS once the national policy is formulated.

9.2 Lessons learnt

- A multichannel approach is desirable to reach WRA with WIFS. The use of institutional set-ups, such as factories and schools, makes it easier to reach WRA. Associating the WIFS programme with an ongoing social development programme in rural areas, and using garment factories as an entry point in urban areas, facilitated programme introduction.

- Social marketing strategies are effective in promoting IFA supplements among rural women and adolescent girls in schools. However, response is better in higher socioeconomic groups.

- Women of low socioeconomic status respond less well, even if WIFS is supplied free of cost. Therefore the strategy for that group needs be modified to increase demand and consumption.

- Creating public awareness through a high-profile launch of the product is important in influencing WRA to buy and consume WIFS.

- An attractive name and a positive image create a more positive attitude towards and demand for the IFA supplement. WIFS for WRA is associated with beauty and health.

- The use of an attractively designed logo, a standardized message and blister packs adds value to the product.

- Establishing the price of IFA supplements in consultation with WRA, for a month's supply of four tablets, aids marketing and ensures that the supplements would be affordable.
- In factory and school situations, a fixed-day approach is effective for the distribution and promotion of IFA tablets.
- Compliance of WIFS was over 70% in unsupervised conditions in rural women and this could be due to an effective social marketing strategy. Key programme factors in the community situation, which possibly play a very positive role, are: effective distribution and availability of IFA, providing training and support for peer counsellors, price regulation, and effective monitoring.
- Adolescent schoolgirls are willing and able to buy WIFS. Knowledge of haemoglobin status is a motivating factor.
- Training quality was reported to be weak and this was attributed to inadequate time being allocated to develop skills for effective counselling
- The production and availability of IEC materials should be ensured prior to the launch of the WIFS programme.
- Simple and standardized monitoring formats are user-friendly and effective. Where a social marketing strategy is used, it is useful to monitor information on the purchase of WIFS, the funds generated, the reasons for discontinuation of WIFS, the reported side-effects and rumours.
- There is a high possibility of rumours damaging the WIFS programme unless timely action is taken. In factories, there was a rumour that the tablets contained amphetamine to make women work harder. Another rumour observed was associating WIFS with contraceptives. Since WIFS is a long-term strategy, it is crucial to be vigilant and to address rumours quickly.
- In factories, women taking WIFS reported positive results. It is important to gather feedback on positive experiences and to build a strategy for promoting WIFS based on the reported benefits of the supplements.
- Rural community women were not as motivated to take WIFS as secondary-school girls. This was possibly due to information on WIFS not being effectively disseminated or the system for regularly accessing tablets being weak.
- Schools are a highly supportive environment to establish practices for preventing iron deficiency and anaemia. Teachers and peer educators play a critical role in influencing adolescent schoolgirls as well as communities. The school-linked programme was effective and should be considered for scaling up to the national level.
- Free distribution, rather than sale of IFA supplements has been proposed for scaling up the programme due to the additional funds required for social marketing.

References

(1) Kanal K, et al. Weekly iron folic acid supplements to prevent anaemia among Cambodian women in three settings: process and outcomes of social marketing and community mobilization. *Nutrition reviews*, December 2005, 63 (12): S126-S133.

(2) Crape BL, et al. Positive impact of a weekly iron folic acid supplement delivered with social marketing to Cambodian women: compliance, participation and haemoglobin levels increase with higher socioeconomic status. *Nutrition reviews*, December 2005, 63 (12): S134-S138.

(3) Longfils P, et al. Weekly iron and folic acid supplementation as a tool to reduce anaemia among primary school children in Cambodia. *Nutrition reviews*, December 2005, 63 (12): S139-S145.

(4) The weekly iron / folate pilot programme for prevention of anaemia in women of reproductive age. Ministry of Health, National Maternal and Child Health Centre, Cambodia, 2001-2002.

(5) Weekly iron folate supplementation, programme evaluation protocol. National Nutrition Programme. September 2007- September 2008.

(6) Tokmoh La-Ong. Personal communication 26th March, 2008. Weekly iron / folate supplementation for secondary school girls in MPA 10 target provinces for 2005-2006.

(7) Tokmoh La-Ong, Personal communication 4th August 2009.

9.3 Cambodia WIFS Programme - A summary

Time framework and coverage	Age group	Anaemia prevalence	Intervention package	Nodal implementing agencies	Impact	Current status
• Phase 1 – March 2001 – Dec 2002. One province 24 000 women in seven garment factories (10 549 women), 139 village communities, five secondary schools. • Phase 2 – 2002, five districts, 371 villages. • Phase 3 – 2008 – five provinces, 78 000 schoolgirls and 33 000 WRAs.	Non-pregnant women. Mean age (years) adolescent girls = 16 years. Garment factory workers = 21 years. Rural village women = 32 years.	47% in WRA and 57% in pregnant women	• WIFS • Nutrition Education	• Ministry of Health	Haemoglobin levels in six months increased significantly (+3.6 g/l) in schoolgirls taking WIFS compared with those not not taking WIFS (+0.8 g/l).	• Government scaled up WIFS programme from January-November 2008, covering 60 000 schoolgirls in five provinces and 33 000 WRAs in one operational district. The intervention package comprised free supply of WIFS and weekly health/nutrition education. • Based on this experience and evaluation analysis, the anaemia prevention programme expected to be launched in 2010.

Supply and consumption of WIFS

Composition, packaging and supply procurement	Cost	Specific approach used	Specific consumption instructions	IFA Supply to recipients		Supervision during WIFS consumption
				Free / purchased	Access	
• Supplied by UNILAB (Manila, Philippines) • Each IFA tablet contained 60 mg of elemental iron and 3.5 mg of folic acid. • Blister packs of four tablets and tertiary packs with 50 small packs. • Package with specially designed logo, standardized message and price. • Name "Red Rose" or "Kolah Korohorm (KK)"	• Selling price of a blister pack of 4 tablets = US$ 0.10. • Estimated cost / beneficiary US $ 5 / WRA for the whole pilot project #	• Fixed day – every Saturday (for factories)	Take supplement at night before sleeping.	• Free to factory workers. • Purchased by WRA in the community. • Women who were considered poor by village community received WIFS free. • Schoolgirls purchased WIFS.	• Team leaders distributed every month to a group of 20-50 women. • Sale of IFA by community person / leader. WIFS sold centrally following monthly village meeting or through door-to-door visit.	• No supervision at factory level since advised to consume WIFS at night. • Consumption of WRA in community or at school not supervised

Cost of the pilot project for 30 000 WRA = apx. US $ 150 000 (excludes cost of IFA tablets) = US $ 5 per WRA

Efforts to increase compliance (IEC / Social mobilization / Strategy)

Positive attributes / benefits experienced	Side-effects reported and managed	Supplement-promotion strategy	Compliance

Benefits reported – sleeping better, feeling stronger. In factories: effort was made to address rumours that tablets were amphetamines to make women work harder or family planning pills or fertility pills. This was done by primarily sharing the positive results experienced by women.	Black faeces, headache, diarrhoea, nausea.	• Social marketing approach used in community and schools. In factories, demand created through organization of counselling and education sessions.
		• Positioned IFA with image of "glowing with good health"; named "Red Rose" in local language – rose associated with beauty and glowing complexion as well as positive self-image. Additional emphasis on freedom from fatigue and tiredness during menstruation.
		  – IEC materials with special logo of a fairy holding a red rose.
		  – Printed materials – posters, stickers, leaflets, billboards, hats and shirts, shoulder bags for girls, mirrors. Logo used on all materials.
		  – Programme launch, mass media usage
		• Social mobilization strategy – small and big launch, lottery programme
		  – IEC counselling by team leaders (factory)
			Varied in different set-ups.
			• 71% WRA in community
			• 57% WRA in factory
			• 55% schoolgirls in secondary school
			• 57.4% in rural villages (higher socioeconomic group)
			• 43.8% rural village WRA (lower socioeconomic group)

Training and monitoring

Training	Monitoring Individual cards / registers etc	Other positive contributing factors
• Training conducted by factory team leaders, community leaders and teachers. Factory team leaders trained in counselling and promotion skills. • Community leaders and teachers trained in skills for promotion and sale of IFA supplements, recording information on monitoring forms and counselling on WIFS and nutrition education. • Manual on WIFS developed and used.	• Factory – standardized monitoring to facilitate analysis and feedback. Forms completed by factory team leaders. • Community monitoring forms completed every three months. Information compiled included supply, purchase, reports of side-effects, rumours, discontinuation and reasons.	• Big launch with involvement of political and religious leaders. • Informing girls of haemoglobin levels motivated and increased compliance.

10. The Philippines

10.1 Scaling Up the WIFS Programme at the national level in partnership with industry

PROJECT AT A GLANCE	
Date of programme	• Phase 1 – 1998 • Phase 2 – 2002 (then discontinued)
Location	• Philippines
Number of participants	• Estimated 30 000 WRA at least 15 years of age (in pilot project)
Project managed by	• Department of Health, in collaboration with the education sector, local government and United Laboratories, Inc. (UNILAB)
Reduction in anaemia rate	• Serum ferritin increased significantly, but minimal change in haemoglobin levels (although hematocrit increased significantly)
Compliance rate	• 95% after 12 months
Programme costs	• Selling price was US$0.28/blister pack of four tablets

A. Project design

Background

A national survey in the Philippines, in 1998, revealed that 50.7% of pregnant women were anaemic and iron deficiency was cited as the most common cause. Major causes of anaemia were low intake of iron-rich foods, the presence of inhibitors in the traditional rice-based diet, low intake of enhancers of iron absorption, vitamin A deficiency, intestinal parasites and, in some regions, malaria. The findings drew attention to the fact that the national programme for prevention of anaemia, launched in 1977, had had very little impact on reducing the public health problem of anaemia during pregnancy. This led to the formulation and implementation of a one-year pilot project that started in November 1998.

Programme goals

The objectives of the project were:

- to introduce preventive supplementation in WRA using community-based social mobilization and communication to promote the new approach (Preventive supplementation would start with a weekly dose of 60 mg of elemental iron and 3.5 mg of folic acid before pregnancy and continue with a weekly dose of 120 mg of elemental iron and 3.5 mg of folic acid when pregnancy was detected.);
- to assess the effectiveness of the combined strategy of social mobilization and WIFS in improving both the knowledge, attitudes and practices, and the iron status of WRA in the project area; and
- to assess the feasibility of taking the programme to scale with WIFS for non-pregnant WRA in the entire country.

Target group and programme roles and responsibilities

The demonstration project, commonly referred to as the Pangasinan Pilot Project, was implemented in three municipalities of Pangasinan Province in northern Luzon: Calasiao, Bimaley and Santa Barbara. The project aimed to cover 30 000 WRA and was implemented by the Government in partnership with the large privately owned local pharmaceutical company, United Laboratories, Inc. (UNILAB). The nodal agency for project implementation was the Department of Health, which collaborated with non-health sectors such as education, local government (mayor and council members) UNILAB. Roles were clearly spelled out. The Department of Health had overall responsibility, while the role of UNILAB was to ensure access to IFA supplements at an agreed, affordable price and to provide support for the social marketing campaigns and monitoring of IFA supplement sales. Monitoring meetings were initially planned every month in the first six months and once every two months thereafter, under the leadership of Department of Health, to discuss progress reports prepared by the health sector in coordination with the school system.

Regular consumption of WIFS was promoted, along with iron-rich food. Social marketing, of which social mobilization was an integral part, was a critical component of the project. Social marketing was positioned around the 4 Ps of marketing:

- Product (the importance of iron and its benefits);
- Price (information on cost and encouragement to buy the product);
- Place (availability of iron tablets at all times) ; and
- Promotion (regarding product, price and place, including advertising, packaging, point-of-sale displays and special events).

The social marketing activities were jointly implemented by the Department of Health and UNILAB. The activities were geared toward developing a new image for iron supplements, promoting the importance of regularly purchasing and consuming WIFS and adoption of this practice by WRA. Women at least 15 years old and who had started menstruating were the primary focus.

IFA supply

The intervention focused on ensuring IFA supply and demand creation. Two iron preparations, both produced by UNILAB, were used, one for non-pregnant women and one for pregnant women. IFA tablets were produced with the following factors in mind: ease of swallowing, size and colour. Elliptically shaped, small tablets were produced in two colours: light pink IFA tablets for non-pregnant women, with a lower dose of iron; and red IFA tablets, with a higher dose of iron, for pregnant women. The name "Femina", highlighting the role of the product in enhancing feminine aspects of the users, was used as the common name for both products. Calling them "Femina 60" and "Femina OB" distinguished the two types. Femina 60 was for weekly consumption by non-pregnant women and contained 60 mg of elemental iron and 3.5 mg of folic acid per tablet. Femina OB was designed for weekly consumption by pregnant women and contained 120 mg of elemental iron and 3.5 mg of folic acid per tablet.

Monitoring meetings were initially planned every month in the first six months and once every two months thereafter, under the leadership of Department of Health, to discuss progress reports prepared by the health sector in coordination with the school system.

Special attention was given to ensuring attractive packaging, since mothers had reported that, in the ongoing national programme, iron supplements were given to women without proper packaging, wrapped in paper, and were thus not viewed as valuable.

The Directorate of Health created a project team to carry out an advisory role during implementation and technical groups were also formed at national as well as municipal levels. Municipalities, with two rural health units, each serving a population of 28 000-36 000 and operating through a network of *barangay* (village) health stations, were put in charge of the overall project, including the supply of iron supplements and their distribution free of charge. Rural health midwives (RHMS) distributed WIFS to pregnant and lactating mothers. These midwives were asked to undertake regular home visits, with the help of *barangay* health and nutrition staff, and also to maintain a record of distribution, consumption and side-effects of WIFS.

Special attention was given to ensuring attractive packaging, since mothers had reported that, in the ongoing national programme, iron supplements were given to women without proper packaging, wrapped in paper, and were thus not viewed as valuable. Four capsules, a month's supply for WRA, were packed in flexible foil to ensure greater stability and protection. These packets were placed in an attractive cover that contained information about the product, food sources of folic acid and iron, product dosage and instructions for use.

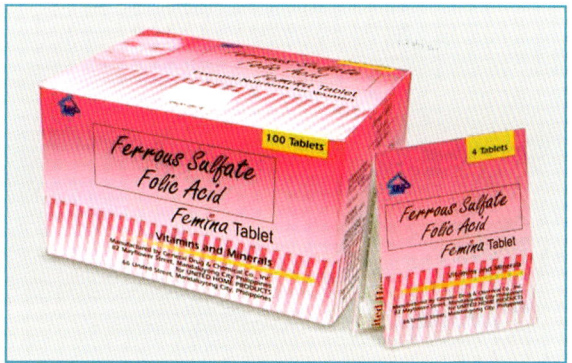

Product shot of Femina tablets

For non-pregnant WRA, WIFS were promoted and marketed for women and their families. The IFA supplements were made available by UNILAB at a fixed cost of 14 Philippine Peso (US$0.28) per package of four tablets. A supply of these tablets was stored with pharmacists as well as with village health workers and at high schools. UNILAB monitored sales by maintaining sales records at drug stores and schools and through village health workers. For pregnant women and those three months postpartum, supplements were provided free and distributed at health centres during visits to rural health workers. A total of 40 tablets were provided free, including 12 tablets given right after delivery. One package of four tablets was given during the monthly check-up. Pregnant woman who failed to go to rural health units were reached by trained *barangay* health workers or midwives responsible for keeping an active list of pregnant and postpartum women and undertaking home visits. Figure 18 presents an overview of the system used for reaching WRA and pregnant mothers.

To promote weekly consumption of IFA, a fixed-day approach was used, with WRA being encouraged to take WIFS every Tuesday night before going to bed. Tuesday was selected as the day for WIFS, since Wednesday was the fixed day for immunization and so health workers would be available to help monitor consumption. Social mobilization activities were accorded high priority, not only to convince women to consume supplements, but also as a means of seeking leadership support from mayors, councillors and priests. Support was also sought from municipal and *barangay* health staff, local storeowners and community residents.

IEC activities

Advocacy and IEC materials included posters, pamphlets, pocket calendars and fliers. The message "Your iron/my iron make us healthy" was used in all the materials. Information promoting Tuesday as WIFS Day was printed on all IEC materials. Guidelines were developed to ensure effective distribution and use of IEC materials by health workers, who were trained to use IEC materials during interpersonal counselling.

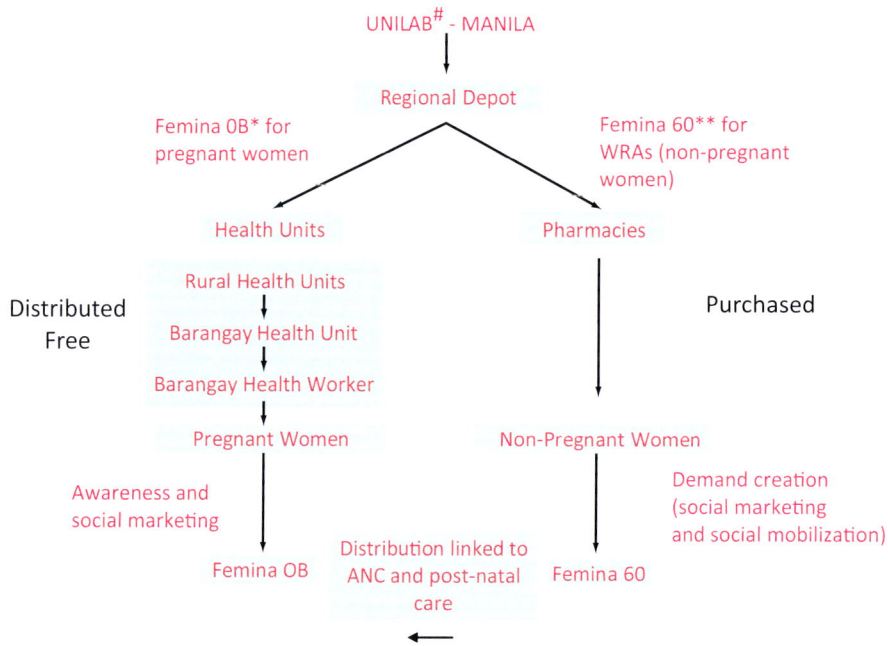

\# Private pharmaceutical company
\#\# Non-pregnant women on becoming pregnant get free supply of Femina OB
* Femina OB - for weekly consumption, contained 120 mg elemental iron and 3.5 mg folic acid per tablet
** Femina 60 - for weekly consumption, contained 60 mg elemental iron and 3.5 mg folic acid per tablet

Interpersonal-communication techniques were used to motivate mothers to regularly attend antenatal services. At every check-up, an appropriate number of IFA tablets and pamphlets on self-care were given to mothers. Cassette tapes, group discussions and other interactive programmes were organized, and general community education programmes were given emphasis to increase the effectiveness of the interpersonal counselling undertaken by health workers. In schools, information campaigns were organized at the municipal and village levels, and billboards, posters and banners were used. A general community education programme, including radio and public address programmes, supported this. Education messages on WIFS were integrated with other health education messages in ongoing health activities. A high-profile launch of the product and intense promotional activities were conducted by UNILAB for target groups in both communities and schools.

Training

Project teams at the national, regional and provincial levels, as well as *barangay* health workers, were trained in social marketing and interpersonal skills. Additionally, prenatal care and service delivery training of all health staff, including midwives at rural health units, included knowledge about iron and IDA, communication skills, project orientation and information regarding their roles and responsibilities. High-school teachers were also trained in various aspects of the project, including interpersonal and counselling skills. All trainers were provided with IEC materials such as posters, primers, fliers and calendars.

Compliance

Purchase and consumption records revealed that over half of the sales of WIFS were from drug stores (56%), followed by sales in health units (31%) and schools (13%). Compliance was high and increased with programme duration, indicating that women accepted WIFS as they became accustomed to taking the pills. By the 12th month of the project, over 95% of respondents indicated that they were taking the supplements.

> Compliance was high and increased with programme duration, indicating that women accepted WIFS as they became accustomed to taking the pills.

Evaluation

The pilot project showed that the use of WIFS is a feasible preventive strategy for controlling anaemia and ensuring sufficient iron reserves before pregnancy in WRA in the Philippines, and an effective alternative to a daily approach.

Figure 19: The impact of the programme was evident from the monitoring of sales records

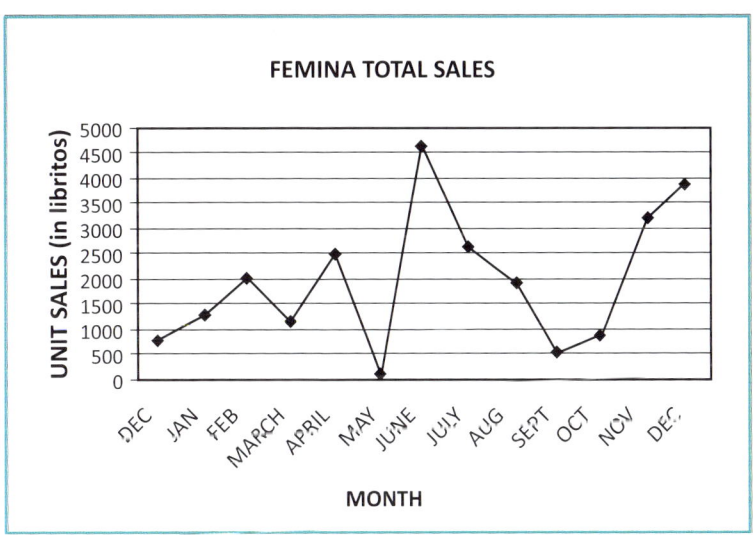

Iron status, as expressed by serum ferritin, significantly improved in both pregnant and non-pregnant women taking WIFS for more than six weeks. However, only a minimal change in haemoglobin was noted, possibly due to a lack of other haeme-forming nutrients. A cut-off point of six weeks for the duration of supplements was selected for two reasons: six weeks was the mid-point of the actual distribution of responses on taking supplements and the period of six weeks resulted in clear–cut group observations with an adequate sample size for comparison.

Surveys were conducted to evaluate the effects of WIFS on haematological parameters in non-pregnant women at baseline and 4.5, 9 and 12 months later. A total of 409 non-pregnant women participated in the study at the time of the baseline survey. The anaemia prevalence at baseline was 33.3%. At the end of 12 months, 359 non-pregnant women were followed up and a highly significant positive effect on serum ferritin levels was reported.

Scaling up

Based on the positive impact of the demonstration project, Femina 60 was launched nationwide in 2002 by the pharmaceutical company producing the supplements, independent of the Department of Health. To promote the use of WIFS, focus was on educating the target market (WRA) and the market influencers of the importance of iron and the implications of iron deficiency. Support and participation was obtained from key persons in local areas, such as village health workers, rural health unit staff, school officials, local government officials and churches. Involvement of teachers was intensified to encourage adolescent girls to take WIFS, and a school programme was part of the national launch.

The communication plan for marketing was a mixture of traditional and non-mainstream media. Education via advertising was given a very high priority and proved effective in creating awareness of IDA and the use of IFA as a preventive measure. The infomercial campaign presented iron deficiency as a potential serial killer victimizing all menstruating women, and used a catch phrase *"Biktima Ka ba?"* ("Are you a victim?"). The second phase of the campaign focused on WIFS as a solution for the "victims". The recall of the dramatic, strong message was enormous among the public. The aim of the campaign was to promote WIFS as a preventive action rather than a therapeutic product. It was observed that a campaign approach was needed to continuously reinforce the importance of women making WIFS a regular habit.

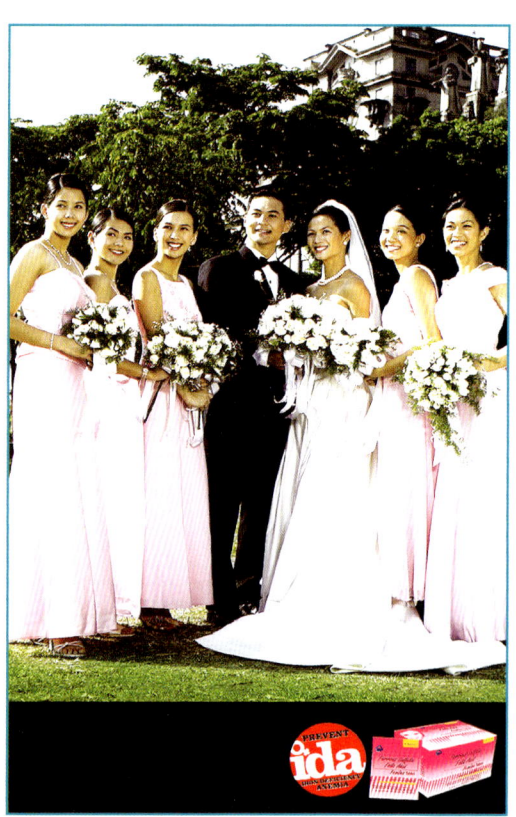

Advertisement used for the launching of the Femina Supplements

Combined strategies of advertising and professional marketing led to high awareness of WIFS, but did not necessarily translate into high usage of Femina. The supplement continued to be perceived, not as a preventive intervention, but as a medicine, since respondents were often looking for clear symptoms that would signal IDA before buying the supplement. In the absence of signs of IDA, WRAs were inclined to believe that they were not susceptible to IDA.

Programme discontinuation

After a few years, UNILAB stopped selling the WIFS supplements and now produces them only upon request for use in specific programmes, usually in other countries. The lack of a lasting national WIFS programme is attributed to a combination of factors:

1. The Department of Health did not adopt a policy on preventive supplementation for anaemia, probably due to the lack of decrease in anaemia rates in the pilot project, despite the very significant increase in ferritin levels. This was possibly also due to insufficient follow-up and discussion with the relevant authorities in the Department. An opportunity to do this was the review of guidelines on micronutrient supplementation that the Department began in mid-2009. The new guidelines include WIFS as a preventive intervention for anaemia in WRA.

2. No studies were conducted after the project to explain why haemoglobin did not increase despite a significant improvement in iron stores in both non-pregnant and pregnant women. Genetic anaemia may be one of the causes, but very little is known about the frequency of such conditions in the Philippines. Inadequate intake of other nutrients, such as vitamin A, vitamin C, and inhibitors of iron absorption may also contribute.

3. The sale of weekly supplements by UNILAB was not as successful as initially hoped, for various reasons: the private sector approach was not supported by a public health campaign to promote the supplements; there was a need for more campaigns and greater advocacy targeting medical doctors and other health workers; the problems in marketing WIFS as a preventive approach, as opposed to a therapeutic supplement for anaemia, were not successfully addressed, and this limited the commercial success of the supplements.

4. One of the underlying problems in promoting interventions to combat anaemia is the fact that symptoms of anaemia are not obvious, at least not until the anaemic person perceives the improved well-being derived from taking supplements. These benefits, which are reported by most women in WIFS programmes, include: feeling more energetic and more productive, having greater concentration, and improved appetite, sleep patterns and menstrual cycles. The promotion of these supplements therefore needs to focus on their ability to improve women's well-being and pregnancy outcomes, even without their being diagnosed as anaemic and iron-deficient.

All of these factors will have to be addressed for WIFS to succeed in the Philippines.

It is important to find ways to reduce anaemia rates, but it is also important to recognize the benefits of improved iron status, even independently of improved haemoglobin, as reported in the literature and by women who take WIFS.

10.2 Lessons learnt

- Social marketing and social mobilization play a major role in creating willingness to purchase WIFS from local government or commercial sources. Social marketing messages should introduce WIFS as part of a healthy lifestyle for WRA.
- Social marketing must cover aspects such as product formulation, product presentation, distribution and marketing activities, which should be in line with government policies.
- A strong public-private partnership is needed for production and marketing of IFA tablets that are safe, reasonably priced and attractive.
- Intense motivation and encouragement from health workers and schoolteachers are required to encourage WRA to buy IFA supplements.
- To promote WIFS, a fixed-day approach is crucial. Selection of the fixed day should take into consideration days that are already fixed for specific intervention actions of other national programmes, such as immunization, so that supportive programme links can be established.
- Availability of WIFS through easily accessible outlets is essential. WIFS should be made widely available for purchase as an over-the-counter supplement in village drugstores or other local stores, including convenience stores (sari-sari stores in the Philippines), health or other development centres and senior schools.
- Development of a communication and social mobilization plan with the involvement of the entire community and with strong support from the authorities, such as local schools and government, results in better ownership of the programme and better acceptance of WIFS by all stakeholders.
- Advocacy and educational activities are more effective when planned and executed with the involvement of medical associations and pharmaceutical companies.
- Uniform and consistent educational messages are essential for promotional activities. IEC materials, developed and used for various promotional activities, should adopt a common look. All IEC materials should contain information on the fixed day for WIFS. In the Philippines, all IEC materials had a basic pink background, a logo bearing the Femina brand name and a single message consistent with the product usage, which positioned IFA as a once-a-week supplement.
- Educational and information activities should comprise interpersonal counselling as well as general community education programmes, such as information campaigns in schools to reinforce messages. Integrating WIFS educational messages with other health education messages is desirable. With an effective communication strategy, compliance tends to increase with programme duration.
- Teachers are credible counsellors, effective in influencing girls to take WIFS. Involvement of schools is critical in reaching WRA in schools and the community.

- Training in social marketing and social mobilization is essential at every level of government, in the health sector and in the education system, as well as for those involved in marketing of drugs. Training should include development of counselling skills.
- To take the WIFS programme to a national scale, the following programme issues must be taken into consideration:
  - A marketing campaign aimed at reminding WRA to take WIFS and encouraging them to develop the habit of taking IFA once a week should be launched. WRA and market influencers should be educated on the importance of preventing anaemia.
  - Schools with adolescent girls can play a very important role.
  - A strong, compelling message on anaemia is needed to encourage regular use of WIFS. Combined strategies of advertising and professional marketing contribute to increased awareness of anaemia.
  - To translate awareness of the importance of WIFS into the practice of regularly purchasing and consuming the supplements, there is a need to emphasize the preventive action of WIFS rather than promoting it as a therapeutic product. This remains a challenge. Efforts are needed to educate WRA and others in the community to recognize symptoms such as dizziness, fatigue and paleness as common symptoms of iron deficiency, and to learn that WIFS can help prevent them.
  - The availability of and easy access to IFA supplements should be ensured. Owners of local drug stores and health staff should be encouraged to become part of the marketing system and direct sellers.
  - People involved in selling WIFS should be equipped with the required information and skills to increase their effectiveness.
  - If WIFS improves iron deficiency but does not reduce anaemia, the causes of this should be investigated while continuing to promote WIFS for the advantage of improved iron status.

References

1. Paulino LS, et al. Weekly iron folic acid supplementation to improve iron status and prevent pregnancy anaemia in Filipino women of reproductive age: The Philippine experience through government and private partnership. *Nutrition reviews*, December 2005, 63 (12): S109-S115.

2. Agdeppa IA, et al. Government industry partnership in weekly iron folic acid supplementation for women of reproductive age in the Philippines: impact on iron status. *Nutrition reviews*, December 2005, 63 (12): S116-S125.

3. Garcia J, Barrett ED, Dizon M. Industry experience in promoting weekly iron folic acid supplementation in the Philippines. *Nutrition reviews*, December 2005, 63 (12): S146-S151.

4. Smitasiri S, Menon A. Strengthening the health of women and children in family planning. *Report of a mission to the Philippines*, May 1998. Manila, WHO Regional Office for the Western Pacific, 1998.

10.3 Philippines WIFS Programme – A summary

Time framework and coverage	Age group	Anaemia prevalence	Intervention package	Nodal implementing agencies	Impact	Current status
• 1998 – one-year pilot project in three municipalities of one province • 2002 – nationwide launch by pharmaceutical company. Discontinued a few years ago since no government policy in place.	WRA at least 15 years of age who had started menstruating.	• Most common cause of anaemia was iron deficiency. • 33% of WRA anaemic. • 50.7% of pregnant women anaemic.	• Social marketing of WIFS. • Promotion of iron-rich food.	• Department of Health, in collaboration with the education sector, local government and a private pharmaceutical company (UNILAB).	• In six weeks, serum ferritin increased significantly, but only minimal change in haemoglobin levels.	• The nationwide programme launched in 2002 was discontinued after a few years since the Department of Health did not adopt a policy on preventive supplementation for anaemia. • Preventive supplementation with WIFS for WRA was included in the revised guidelines on micronutrient supplementation, developed in 2009.

Supply and consumption of WIFS

Composition, packaging and supply procurement	Cost	Specific approach used	Specific consumption instructions	IFA Supply to recipients		Supervision during WIFS consumption
				Free / purchased	Access	
Produced by UNILAB. Two types* Light pink – Femina 60 (for non-pregnant WRA), elemental iron = 60 mg, folic acid = 3.5 mg. Red – Femina OB (for pregnant women), elemental iron = 120 mg, folic acid = 3.5 mg. Elliptically shaped small tablets, attractively packed in flexible foil * both for weekly consumption.	Selling cost of tablet US$ 0.28 for a blister pack of four tablets.	• Fixed-day approach. Tuesday selected as WIFS day since the next day was the fixed day for immunization and could help in monitoring by health workers team.	Take supplement at night before sleeping.	• Purchased by WRA (non-pregnant) at the agreed price of US$ 0.28 for four tablets. • Free distribution only for pregnant women and for three months postpartum. Total of 40 IFA tablets free – of which 12 tablets provided right after delivery.	• WIFS supplements for sale to WRA (non-pregnant) stored with pharmacists, village health workers and high schools. • Pregnant women handed WIFS tablets during routine check-up. Pregnant women not going to health units reached through home visits by midwives or health workers.	• Not supervised

Cost of the pilot project for 30 000 WRA = apx. US $ 150 000 (excludes cost of IFA tablets) = US $ 5 per WRA

Efforts to increase compliance (IEC / Social mobilization / Strategy)

Positive attributes / benefits experienced	Side-effects reported and managed	Supplement-promotion strategy	Compliance
Emphasis on WIFS and "making healthy"	• No significant difference in frequency of side-effects between daily and weekly supplements. • Acceptance of WIFS was high with increased duration in consumption.	• High-profile launch and intensive promotional activities. • Social marketing of IFA tablets – four principles of social marketing applied. • IEC materials included posters, pamphlets, calendars, fliers. • Specific main message "Your iron / my iron make us healthy". Linked to health education sessions or messages. • Interpersonal communication technique to increase response of mothers. • Cassette tapes, group discussions and other interactive programmes organized. • Social mobilization accorded high priority – to convince women, as well as a means of seeking leadership support from political leaders, policy-makers, religious leaders, health sector staff, and local store owners. • Information campaign organized at village level using billboards, posters and banners. General community education – radio and public address programme • Involvement of teachers and education through advertisements was intensified. WIFS was positioned as a preventive intervention and not a medicine.	• In pilot phase compliance of WIFS increased with time. By 12th month over 95% of respondents indicated taking WIFS. • In nationwide launch, WIFS continued to be viewed as a medicine. UNILAB stopped selling WIFS after a few years.

Training and monitoring

Training	Monitoring Individual cards / registers etc	Other positive contributing factors
• Project teams at national, regional, provincial levels were trained in social marketing. • Knowledge about iron and anaemia built into training of antenatal and postnatal workers. • Health workers trained on skills for interpersonal counselling and usage of IEC materials. • High-school teachers trained on various aspects of projects, interpersonal counselling skills. • Training materials comprised posters, primers, flier fans, calendars. • Guidelines for health workers to ensure effective distribution and coverage of all IEC materials.	• UNILAB monitored sales by maintaining sales records at drug stores, schools and village health workers • Health workers maintained a record of distribution, consumption and side-effects of WIFS.	• Creation of a project team and a technical team. • Active role of private-sector pharmaceutical agency.

Annexes

Annex 1 : Documentation of process and impact of selected case studies on preventive weekly IFA supplementation (WIFS) for women of reproductive age (WRA)

Template used for country case studies

The template included the following key features of the programme:

1. Basic strategy and action plan of the WIFS programme.
2. Programme goals, objectives, strategy, targets, intervention package and distribution channel(s).
3. IFA tablet composition, supply, cost, distribution, storage, administration and overall logistical management.
4. Enabling components of the programme: information, education and communication (IEC) and social mobilization activities with special reference to efforts to address the issues of compliance, management, training and capacity-building, monitoring and supervision.
5. Progress and impact.
6. Cost and programme sustainability.
7. Policy implications in the region.

Intervention details for various programme components		
Programme issues	A. Project / Programme coverage, Goals/ Objectives	Analysis / Comments

<ul><li>Pilot effort / project / scaled up district / state / national programme</li><li>Coverage – (cluster of villages / block/ district/ national / any other) – specific details of population (in millions) covered</li><li>Implementation period</li><li>Age group
  - Adolescents
  - WRA (both adolescents and women > 19 years)</li><li>Any other</li></ul>		

	B. Project strategies	
<ul><li>Intervention package (WIFS alone or a packaged approach with deworming / family-life education / any other)</li><li>Reaching the target – built on ongoing health programmes, non-health programmes such as education or any other</li><li>Nodal sector responsible identified– Government (Health sector and non-health sector) / NGO / private sector / pharmaceutical sector/ institution</li><li>Programme partners identified (health / non-health sector, private sector, pharmaceutical sector / any other).</li><li>Roles and responsibilities defined and agreed</li></ul>		

	C. Advocacy and political commitment

- Situation analysis of WRA (iron / anaemia status, dietary habits (knowledge, attitudes, practices influencing iron status)– available / undertaken
- Advocacy activities
  - Advocacy support materials developed
  - Advocacy meeting organized for sensitization and seeking of commitment from policy-makers
  - High-profile launch
- Information on WIFS issued by the nodal department in charge of implementation

	D. Management of project / programme

- Operational plan or working document developed (with or without the involvement of stakeholders)
- Time-frame
- Specific project team formed linked to nodal sector
- Special effort made to involve community leaders / community groups / any other
- Management team at different levels – District Steering Committee / Community Health Committee / any other

	E. Ensuring IFA supply – Procurement and provision or channels for reaching target group

- Product specified
  - Form (tablet / capsule)
  - Composition of tablet / capsule
  - Coated / non-coated
  - Packaging (blister / flexible foil)
  - No. of tablets per pack
  - Colour (rationale, if any, for selection of colour)
- Estimating requirement
  - Centralized – calculated based on population and coverage
  - Decentralized (at village / block / district/ state level) and forwarded to nodal department
- Procurement organized
  - Government procurement
  - UNICEF supply
  - Private sector contribution
  - Any other
- Nodal organization responsible for ensuring timely supply
  - Government (sector),
  - Non- government,
  - Any other
- Supply channel defined
  - Central to state to district or cluster of villages / any other

- Storage facility identified
  - Village-level depot, Shops / pharmaceutical centres, health centres, schools / education centres, Nutrition programme or other development programme,
  - Any other
- Distribution channel for IFA supplements
  - Existing delivery system for IFA to pregnant women studied to strategize distribution channel
  - Health sector channel (traditional)
  - Linkage with ongoing health programme
  - Non-health sector (non-traditional)
  - Private pharmaceutical sector
  - Any other
- Strategy for reaching beneficiaries (traditional / non-traditional)
  - Handing over of supplements directly to beneficiaries or WRA (free supply) by (village health workers, non-health village workers, teachers, factory supervisors / factory group leaders, voluntary workers – girl-to-girl or woman-to-woman approach)
  - Ensuring beneficiaries informed where and how (purchase or free) to access IFA supplement (community centres, health sector / non-health sector depots, factories, schools, sale depots, general market system, WRA / girls' clubs / groups
  - Ensuring consumption and high compliance
  - Fixed-day approach
  - Specific instructions regarding time of consumption
  - Specific instructions on precautions regarding IFA consumption (e.g. following full meals, not on empty stomach, before retiring at night, avoiding tea / coffee prior to or after WIFS, usage of water for swallowing)
  - Monitoring compliance
  - Supervised / unsupervised consumption
  - Compliance card (individual) introduced
  - Compliance register (individual / group/ class) introduced

F. Demand creation for WIFS

- Qualitative study and identification of resistance points
- Development of special message to create positive image of iron tablets
- Effort to dispel any rumour / suspicion
- Specific focus on increasing compliance and addressing the problem of side-effects
- Social marketing and promotion of product for purchase by community
  - Creation of special logo
  - Creation of support materials
- Development and production of IEC support materials

G. Capacity-building / training

- Training plan (levels and persons trained)
- Training manual
- Focus of training

	H. Establishment of monitoring system
<ul><li>Monitoring programme operations (IEC, training, supply, management of intervention)</li><li>Monitoring supply of supplements Timely supply at state / district level, Timely supply available for beneficiaries</li><li>Monitoring individual and group compliance and consumption<ul><li>Individual cards, group registers</li><li>Any other</li></ul></li><li>Strengthening "feedback" mechanisms<ul><li>Coordination committee / meetings (frequency)</li><li>Village / block district meetings</li><li>Monthly / quarterly reports</li></ul></li></ul>	
	I. Evaluation
<ul><li>Baseline survey undertaken</li><li>Process – lessons learnt prior to scaling up, including determinants of compliance, sustainability factors</li><li>Impact – on knowledge, attitudes, practices; Hb levels; and iron status</li></ul>	
	J. Budget / resources
<ul><li>Financial (government funding, -international funding)</li><li>Cost per beneficiary</li></ul>	
	K. Scaling up WIFS intervention / policy implications
<ul><li>Lessons learnt, documented and intervention scaled up</li><li>Current status<ul><li>Administrative order or intervention guidelines issued</li><li>Incorporation in state / national policy</li></ul></li></ul>	

Annex 2 : The Recommendations of the WHO Global Expert Consultation on Weekly Iron and Folic Acid Supplementation for Preventing Anaemia in Women of Reproductive Age

are available at

http://www.who.int/nutrition/publications/micronutrients/weekly_iron_folicacid.pdf

Updated versions of these guidelines can be found in the WHO Nutrition website, at http://www.who.int/nutrition/en/

WEEKLY IRON-FOLIC ACID SUPPLEMENTATION (WIFS) IN WOMEN OF REPRODUCTIVE AGE: ITS ROLE IN PROMOTING OPTIMAL MATERNAL AND CHILD HEALTH

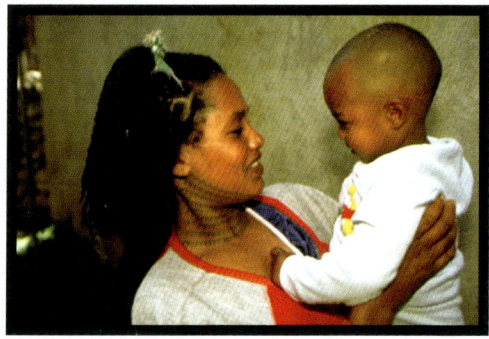

PURPOSE

This position statement is based on the consensus of a World Health Organization (WHO) Global Consultation on Weekly Iron and Folic Acid Supplementation (WIFS) for Preventing Anaemia in Women of Reproductive Age held in Manila, Philippines, 25-27 April 2007 and summarizes recommendations based on a desk review commissioned by the WHO Regional Office for the Western Pacific (WPRO) and additional evidence presented and discussed in the expert consultation. It is intended for a wide audience including program implementing partners, scientists and governments involved in the design and implementation of micronutrient programs as public health interventions.

BACKGROUND

Anaemia is a multi-factorial disorder that requires a multi-pronged approach for its prevention and treatment. Iron deficiency and infections are the most prevalent etiological factors. However other conditions may have a contributory role. They include nutritional deficiencies of vitamin A, vitamin B12, folate and riboflavin as well as thalassemias and hemoglobinopathies. The global prevalence of anemia is estimated to be 30.2% in non-pregnant women rising to 47.4% during pregnancy (de Benoist B et al, 2008). Weekly iron supplementation, in synchrony with the turnover of mucosal cells, has been proposed as a more efficient preventive approach in public health programs (Viteri FE, 1995; Viteri FF et al 1998). The approach is attractive because side effects are thought to be less prominent, and it may be both operationally easier to manage at the community level and more sustainable over extended time periods. Improving iron and folate nutrition of women of reproductive age could improve pregnancy outcomes as well as enhance maternal and infant health. The prudent pragmatic approach is therefore considered to be the recommendation of WIFS in appropriately selected settings where the necessary program monitoring is feasible. Additional short-term efficacy trials are unlikely to provide more useful information about potential long-term effectiveness. The findings of the first three pilot projects were reviewed at a previous meeting held at WPRO in October 2003, a report of which is available on the WPRO website (www.wpro.who.int). The findings, conclusions and recommendations of these projects were published in a supplement of the international journal Nutrition Reviews, December 2005, (II)S95 S108. To date, more than 30 papers have been published globally, reporting findings, conclusions and recommendations on the use of the WIFS approach for the prevention of iron deficiency and anaemia.

THE WHO GLOBAL EXPERT CONSULTATION

A WHO Global Expert Consultation on Weekly Iron and Folic Acid Supplementation for Preventing Anaemia in Women of Reproductive Age was convened in Manila, Philippines in 2007 to discuss the findings of a desk review and discuss the public health implications of the results, especially in developing countries. The consultation objectives included a formal assessment of the review, an analysis of all available evidence related to efficacy, effectiveness, safety and feasibility of preventive supplementation with WIFS programs in improving iron and folate status before and during the early months of pregnancy, a discussion on specific conditions under which WIFS may be implemented effectively and are most likely to have a significant impact on iron and folic acid status before and during pregnancy, and the identification and prioritization of knowledge gaps for which additional research is needed. The proceedings of the consultation, including conclusions and recommendations by the participants, are expected to be published in a special supplement of the Food and Nutrition Bulletin in 2009.

WEEKLY IRON AND FOLIC ACID SUPPLEMENTATION

WIFS is an approach that can be effective for ensuring adequate iron status of women, particularly before pregnancy and during the first trimester in communities where food-based strategies are not yet fully implemented or effective.

Short-and medium-term WIFS has been effective in reducing the prevalence of anaemia among women of reproductive age in several community settings where the necessary support, social marketing and interpersonal advocacy ensured adequate compliance.

Although the proven method for decreasing the risk for neural tube defects (NTDs) is through daily dosing with folic acid before pregnancy through the first trimester of pregnancy, WIFS provides an additional opportunity for ensuring adequate folate status before pregnancy and in the very early stages of pregnancy particularly for those who may become pregnant or do not know that they are already pregnant and are not covered by other programs. Many pregnancies are not planned. Various studies have demonstrated that WIFS can improve iron status in women of reproductive age when supplementation is continuous for periods from several months to two years (Beaton GH, McCabe GP, 1999). A current review (Margetts B, 2007) concluded that WIFS taken for at least 12 weeks improved iron status, as judged by increased hemoglobin and in some studies serum ferritin levels. The impact of weekly supplementation with 60 mg of iron was similar to daily supplementation except in severely anaemic women.

CONSULTATION RECOMMENDATIONS

The recommendations summarized here below represent the conclusions of the experts in the consultation.

- Strategies to combat both iron deficiency and anaemia, and to improve iron reserves and folate status in women of reproductive age should be integrated. Deworming, measures to prevent hookworm infections, the promotion of improved bioavailable iron intake, as well as interventions to control other prevalent causes of anemia, particularly malaria and other infections, and vitamin A deficiency need to be considered.

- In population groups where the prevalence of anaemia is above 20% among women of reproductive age and mass fortification programs of staple foods with iron and folic acid are unlikely to be implemented within 1-2 years, WIFS should be considered as a strategy for the prevention of iron deficiency, the improvement of pre-pregnancy iron reserves and the improvement of folate status in some women. If data on anaemia prevalence in women of reproductive age is not available, anaemia prevalence in other groups such as pregnant women (>40% anaemia prevalence) or children under 5 years of age may be used as a proxy. In the absence of such information, criteria such as dietary patterns and socioeconomic status may be considered. Women from low income groups who may not have access to processed iron-fortified food products and other sources of highly bioavailable iron could be considered a priority group for this intervention.

- The weekly supplement should contain 60 mg iron in the form of ferrous sulphate ($FeSO_4 \cdot 7H_2O$) and 2800 µg folic acid, although evidence for the effective dose of folic acid for weekly supplementation is very limited. Daily folic acid supplementation is effective for reducing the risk of NTDs (Botto LD et al, 1999). The recommendation for the weekly folic acid dosage is based on the participants' rationale of providing 7 times the recommended daily dose to prevent NTDs and the limited experimental evidence demonstrating that this dose can improve red blood cell folate concentrations to levels that have been associated with a reduced risk for NTDs. The iron dose recommended for WIFS may cause short-term gastrointestinal discomfort and black stool, but there is no reported risk of long-term toxicity. The participants also agreed that the recommended weekly folic acid dose has no known toxicity, although evidence for this was limited. Two published studies evaluating weekly folic acid supplementation were considered. In Mexico, women received 5.0 mg folic acid for 3 months, and their red blood cell folate levels were still in the range associated with a 50% lower risk of NTDs one week after the last tablet was consumed (Martinez-de Villarreal LE et al, 2001). They also showed a 50% decrease in the incidence of anencephaly and spina bifida cases, and a significant reduction in infant mortality and disability after two years (Martinez-de Villarreal LE et al, 2002). In New Zealand, a once a week supplement of 2.8 mg of folic acid taken for 12 weeks increased women's red blood cell folic acid levels to concentrations associated with a reduced risk of bearing a child with a NTD (Norsworthy B et al 2004).

- Two situations may necessitate supplementation with iron alone. Fortification of staple foods with folic acid has been shown to be very effective and is being widely implemented. Iron alone should be used in weekly supplementation programs where mandatory folic acid fortification has been introduced and shown to be effective if fortification with iron has not been implemented or is ineffective. Antifolate antimalarial treatment is employed in some malaria endemic regions. There is some evidence to suggest that the efficacy of these drugs may be reduced by folic acid supplementation. In these settings, it is considered prudent to provide iron only weekly supplements.

- Upon confirmation of pregnancy, women should receive standard antenatal care. The current WHO recommendation is to provide daily supplementation with 60 mg iron and 400 ug folic acid to women during pregnancy and the first 3 months postpartum.

- WIFS programs must be integrated with other efforts to control iron deficiency and anaemia and should be planned as long-term self-sustained interventions that women of reproductive age will utilize during their childbearing years.

- Successful implementation of WIFS programs will require motivation and creation of demand by women of reproductive age as the starting point for promoting this new approach, establishing adequate mechanisms to start and sustain programs, including adequate funding, community level support and public-private partnerships including nongovernmental organizations, an uninterrupted supply of good quality iron and folic acid supplements, the development and implementation of effective communication strategies with the media and other information channels, establishment of methods for promoting compliance by women of reproductive age, especially when consumption is not supervised, and integration with effective existing delivery systems in health, education and the private sector (e.g. in factories, markets, and local shops) as well as through community organizations.

- Baseline data are needed before launching WIFS interventions; programs must be monitored closely with regard to both processes and outcomes, during the first year, and then annually for the first 5 years. Monitoring and evaluation systems should be implemented to determine if the intended outcomes are being achieved.

SUMMARY OF STATEMENT DEVELOPMENT

This statement was prepared by the WHO Department of Nutrition for Health and Development in close collaboration with the Regional Office for the Western Pacific (WPRO). Dr. Juan Pablo Pena-Rosas (WHO) and Dr. Luca Tommaso Cavalli-Sforza (WPRO) summarized the conclusions and recommendations. This position statement is based on background documents, including a desk review commissioned to Professor Barrie Margetts and his team at the School of Public Health, University of Southampton (United Kingdom) in 2007 by WPRO. This review included all published work done on WIFS in women of reproductive age to better define the potential benefits of WIFS in preparing women of reproductive age for pregnancy. All available information related to WIFS was discussed at a global consultation held at WPRO jointly with WHO Headquarters in Manila, Philippines in 2007. The desk review provided the updated background for the expert consultation discussions. Studies considered in the review were identified through searching key databases, contacts with principal investigators, and contacts with a number of organisations and agencies that have been gathering literature in the relevant areas of work. Studies were a mix of efficacy and effectiveness designs. This was followed by four invited written commentaries by experts in the fields of iron and folic acid metabolism and public health. In making the recommendations, additional information gathered at the consultation was considered in conjunction with conclusions drawn from the review of both controlled and uncontrolled studies. The consensus conclusions and recommendations from the consultation were revised and summarized for this statement.

CONFLICTS OF INTEREST

All participants in the consultation were asked to submit and sign a Declaration of Interest statement which are on file. There were no known conflicts of interest disclosed among the participants and those developing this statement.

PLANS FOR UPDATE

It is anticipated that the recommendations in this position statement will remain valid until December 2010. The Department of Nutrition for Health and Development at WHO Headquarters in Geneva will be responsible for initiating a review following formal WHO Handbook for Guideline Development procedures at that time.

REFERENCES

de Benoist B et al., eds. Worldwide prevalence of anaemia 1993-2005. WHO Global Database on Anaemia. Geneva, World Health Organization, 2008 (http://whqlibdoc.who.int/publications/2008/9789241596657_eng.pdf, accessed 3 February 2009).

Viteri FE et al. True absorption and retention of supplemental iron is more efficient when iron is administered every three days rather than daily to iron-normal and iron-deficient rats. Journal of Nutrition, 1995, 125:82-91.

Viteri FE. A new concept in the control of iron deficiency: community-based preventive supplementation of at-risk groups by the weekly intake of iron supplements. Biomedical and Environmental Sciences, 1998, 11:46-60.

Beaton GH, McCabe GP. Efficacy of intermittent iron supplementation in the control of iron deficiency anemia in developing countries: An analysis of experience. Ottawa, The Micronutrient Initiative, 1999.

Margetts BM, Tallant A, Armstrong E. Weekly iron and folic acid supplementation for women of reproductive age: a review of published studies. Desk review prepared for WPRO. 2007.

Botto LD et al. Neural-tube defects. New England Journal of Medicine, 1999, 341:1509-19.

Martinez de Villarreal LE et al. [Impact of weekly administration of folic acid on folic acid blood levels]. Salud Pública de México, 2001, 43:103-107.

Martinez de Villarreal L et al. Decline of neural tube defects cases after a folic acid campaign in Nuevo Leon, Mexico. Teratology, 2002, 66:249-256.

Norsworthy B et al. Effects of once-a-week or daily folic acid supplementation on red blood cell folate concentrations in women. European Journal of Clinical Nutrition, 2004, 58:548-554.

SUGGESTED CITATION

WHO. Weekly iron–folic acid supplementation (WIFS) in women of reproductive age: its role in promoting optimal maternal and child health. Position statement. Geneva, World Health Organization, 2009 (http://www.who.int/nutrition/publications/micronutrients/weekly_iron_folicacid.pdf, accessed [date]).

FOR FURTHER INFORMATION, PLEASE CONTACT:

Department of Nutrition for Health and Development (NHD)
World Health Organization
20, Avenue Appia, 1211 Geneva, Switzerland
Email: micronutrients@who.int
WHO home page: http://www.who.int

Annex 3 : Criteria for ensuring the quality of iron and folic acid supplement tablets

(from the Recommendations of the WHO Global Consultation on Weekly Iron and Folic Acid Supplementation for Preventing Anaemia in Women of Reproductive Age, Manila, Philippines, 25-27 April 2007)

The following should be considered to ensure a quality product attractive to women of reproductive age:

1. Tablet quality
    - Tablets should be rapidly soluble in the stomach, even in the presence of a meal.
    - Tablets should be film-coated to be tasteless and odourless and to limit gastric side-effects.
    - A quality assurance programme must be in place for the long term.

2. Appropriate storage
    - Store at temperatures not exceeding 30° C and with low humidity if possible.
    - Secure storage to avoid risk of accidental ingestion by children.

3. Packaging and design of supplements has important implications for:
    – maintenance of quality e.g. blister/flexifoil to prevent moisture;
    – compliance e.g. colour, attractiveness of packaging, messages/branding, coating; and
    – safety e.g. number in pack, not sugar-coated (to avoid accidental consumption by children).

4. The number of supplements per pack should be decided at country level, taking the distribution system and safety into consideration
    – For example, four tablets per pack for monthly distribution is safer but more expensive.
    – 26 tablets are enough for six months and thus require less contact and this reduces the packaging cost, but may be less safe due to risk of accidental ingestion by children.
    – A blister pack of 26 WIFS tablets can be combined with one mebendazole tablet where deworming every six months is recommended.

5. Formative research is needed to determine the best way to present supplements to optimize compliance.

Annex 4 : Indicators for establishing, monitoring and evaluating programmes

(from the Recommendations of the WHO Global Consultation on Weekly Iron and Folic Acid Supplementation for Preventing Anaemia in Women of Reproductive Age, Manila, Philippines, 25-27 April 2007)

Baseline	Six months / annually	
	Impact	
Biological assays	Sources	Indicators
• Haemoglobin • Serum ferritin • Soluble transferrin receptor • C-reactive protein[1] • α-1 acid glycoprotein • Red cell folate • Serum folate • Serum vitamin B12	• Haemoglobin • Serum ferritin • Soluble transferrin receptor • C-reactive protein[1] • α-1 acid glycoprotein • Red cell folate • Serum folate	• National/subnational statistics • Delivery sites / community organizations / hospital / maternity homes • Paediatric services	• Maternal anaemia prevalence • Maternal iron deficiency prevalence • Maternal morbidity / mortality • Gestational age at birth • Birth weight • Stillbirths • Neonatal / infant mortality • NTDs • Prevalence of anaemia in infants at ~6 months

[1] C-reactive protein and α-1 acid glycoprotein are alternative acute phase markers for excluding high ferritin values due to inflammation or infection from survey data.